Easy for You to Say

Easy for You to Say

Q&As for Teens Living with Chronic Illness or Disability

MIRIAM KAUFMAN, M.D.

3RD EDITION
REVISED AND UPDATED

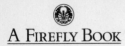

A FIREFLY BOOK

Published by Firefly Books Ltd. 2012

Publisher Cataloging-in-Publication Data (U.S.)
Kaufman, Miriam.
Easy for you to say : Q and As for teens living with chronic illness or disabilities / Miriam Kaufman.
3rd ed., rev., updated, expanded.
[320] p. : col. photos. ; cm.
Includes index.
Summary: Profiles of challenged youth as they address issues including: family, doctors and medical issues, friends and dating, school and work, alcohol and street drugs, medications and sexuality.
ISBN-13: 978-1-77085-099-6 (pbk.)
1. Chronic diseases in adolescence. 2. Teenagers with disabilities – Conflict of life. I. Title.
362.196008 dc23   RJ380.K385 2012

Library and Archives Canada Cataloguing in Publication
Kaufman, Miriam
Easy for you to say : q & a's for teens living with chronic illness or disability / Miriam Kaufman. -- 3rd ed.
 Includes index.
ISBN 978-1-77085-099-6
1. Chronic diseases in adolescence--Miscellanea.
2. Teenagers with disabilities--Conduct of life. I. Title.
RJ380.K38 2012   362.19600835   C2012-901993-3

Printed in Canada.

The publisher gratefully acknowledges the financial support for our publishing program by the Government of Canada through the Canada Book Fund as administered by the Department of Canadian Heritage.

Contents

Preface

Many teens and young adults have what are now called "special health care needs," what many of us think of as a chronic illness or disability. If you are reading this book, you are probably one of them.

I have the really great job of meeting with young people and talking with them about how their condition affects their lives and their place in their family and in the world. They talk to me about how they feel about their bodies, how they relate to people their age, school issues, drugs and alcohol, medications, moving to adult care, learning how to drive, their worries and many more topics.

I wrote the first edition of this book a long time ago. The world has changed and my patients ask me more and more interesting questions, so I have updated it. I could have written a book just for people with cystic fibrosis or lupus or seizures or transplants, but I decided instead to write for everyone who is living with a chronic illness or disability. I didn't want to separate people into little compartments. Teens with long-term conditions have a lot in common. They also have lots in common with teens who are not affected by any medical problem. In fact, you are more like other teens than you are different from them.

The questions in this book (it is in a question/comment/complaint-and-answer format) come from teens I met with while researching the book, from my patients and from colleagues all over the world. Some are combinations of questions asked by several kids. In all cases, I've been careful to make sure that the identity of the person who asked the question remains confidential, sometimes by even changing the condition, if it doesn't change the context of the question. So don't look only for questions from people who have the same condition as you—you might miss other questions and answers that are relevant to you also. Having said that, the book is organized in such a way that you don't have to start at the beginning and read every question in order. Skip around and read a question here and another there, if you like—though it wouldn't be a bad thing to read each chapter from beginning to end, either.

Because I think that attitude has a big impact on how disabling any condition is, some readers may feel I have a Pollyanna-type approach to problems. I don't want to minimize how difficult it can be to be singled out as different when you are an adolescent. But I also know that many young people with what are considered to be serious diseases or disabilities live regular lives and do regular things.

You may also have problems with my strong belief in fighting for what you need and want. My answers may involve suggestions to write letters, send emails, make phone calls, and be an advocate or even an activist. I try to provide alternatives for people who don't want to try these things, but I do think that fighting for what you need often works—and helps you feel in control and powerful.

I wasn't a teen with a chronic illness or disability. I got my chronic condition much later in life (when I was 31), so there is no way I can understand completely what you are going through. On the other hand, as a teen I was an outcast for other reasons, I know what it is like to have a health condition as an adult and I have spent my whole career talking with teens about their concerns.

I asked the teenagers I met with when writing this book what they would like to say to a teen who has just found out that he or she has a serious condition. I got answers like "Just look around when you are in the hospital; you'll realize it could be worse," "Show your parents and doctors that you're capable, then tell them—not the other way around," "You are going to gain respect for other people like you never had before," "If doctors and nurses are getting on your nerves, let them know," "Don't be scared, just go with it" and "You are still the same person you were."

As far as I'm concerned, these teens are the real experts.

Acknowledgments

THIS BOOK HAS A LONG HISTORY, and I have thanked many people who helped me with the first two editions in those books. I am still very grateful to all of them, but don't want half the book to be acknowledgments, so I will just say "thanks" to all of you who helped in so many ways.

The world has changed since I wrote the first edition and I have had help from many people to keep the book relevant and up-to-date. An army of teens, nurse-practitioners, nurses, psychologists, doctors and social workers sprang into action when I sent out an urgent plea to reread the last edition and give me advice. They include Anjali Aggarwal, Ping Chiang, Arlene Chaves, Arlette Lefebvre, Brenda Reid, Cathy Daniels, Danielle Ruskin, Grace Martin, Janette Reyes, Jennifer Tyrrell, Kathy Martin and Krista Keilty. Nadya Nalli spent hours reviewing and updating the medications in Appendix 2, such that she is now a coauthor on that part of the book.

Geraldine Cullen-Dean, Andrea Regina and Karen Sappleton not only reviewed the last edition and made many suggestions, they supported me with chocolate and good humor, and any eye rolling was done behind my back. Khush Amaria and Sharon Lorber weren't able to back me up on this one, as they were busy with their new babies, but I know they would have and they support me in many other ways. Chocolate and good humor also came from Gillian Thompson, Cathy Maser and Nicole Gibson. My sidekick Ian Chen was always there, often doing stuff I should have done so that I could write.

I am very grateful to Firefly Books. This book wouldn't have happened if Key Porter hadn't published the first and second editions, but when they went under in 2011, I thought this book was gone forever. Firefly jumped in and offered to publish an updated version of the book. Young people were telling me that the book was useful to them but was missing important information, especially related to electronics and the interconnected world we all live in today. I am very happy that Firefly was willing to make this new edition a reality so that E4U2S continues to be a support for young people around the world.

1 Family Relationships

MOST OF YOU LIVE WITH YOUR FAMILIES. Whether you are close to them or not, whether you are dependent on family members for daily care or not, they have a big impact on your life. Even if you don't live at home, your family (even if you never see them) still influences you. As you get older, you will create your own family. It may include people you are biologically related to (including your own children) and may extend to other people you care about.

> I go to most of my appointments at the hospital on my own (I'm 16). Last week I had an exam at school and totally forgot a clinic appointment. My father has taken away my phone for a month as a punishment (he's letting my little brother use it!). I need my phone. How can I get it back?

I guess your father is hoping that if there is a big punishment, you won't forget any more appointments. And it sounds like he is pretty mad that you missed it. He might have to pay a fee for a missed appointment, or maybe it was a referral you had been waiting a long time for. Or it could be that he has gotten used to you being more responsible for your care and is worried that he is going to have to become more involved again.

Whatever the reason, I suggest that you ask to meet with him to discuss a plan for remembering your clinic appointments. Figure out ahead of time how you want to manage this.

You might use the calendar on your phone to keep track of all your commitments, and set the alarm function to remind you the evening before and the morning of your appointments. You will need to commit to putting your next appointment in your calendar when it is booked. You should make sure that your main team at the hospital has your number so that if there are changes they can get in touch with you. You might want to offer to show your dad your next appointment in your calendar the day it is booked so that he can see you are keeping your end of the bargain.

It would also be smart to address some of the reasons why he might be upset. Acknowledge that you understand why he is worried about this and perhaps offer to pay any fee charged for a missed appointment.

If he agrees to the plan, you'll need your phone for it, so that should solve your problem—and get you to the hospital when you are supposed to be there.

I am 13. Last week a couple of new friends from my school were at my house. We went to the kitchen to get a snack and my mother came in and said, "Didn't you have your snack already?" and then said to my friends, "She's diabetic, you know. She has to watch what she eats and when she eats it." I was so embarrassed! How can I persuade her not to do this again?

Parents get used to being in control of their kids' lives, including their illnesses, when their children are young. Now that you are growing up and are ready to take more control, it's hard for your mother to adjust to this. It could also be that she's been worried about your diabetic control and somehow thought it would help to mention your diabetes to your friends.

The first thing you need to do is assess how much responsibility you are taking for your illness. Do you test your blood without being reminded? Do you inject your insulin yourself? When you are running low on insulin, syringes or other diabetic paraphernalia, do you let someone know, rather than just waiting for your mother to notice?

If you are doing all these things, sit down with your mother and point out to her that your diabetes is your disease, that you are taking much of the responsibility for it and that it is up to you to decide when to tell friends about it.

If you aren't yet in charge of your diabetes, you can still let your mother know that it was embarrassing for you and that you like to know people a bit better before they find out you have a chronic condition. You can also take the opportunity to make a plan with her for taking over your own basic care.

My sister, who is a year older than I am, often makes mean comments about my illness and how I look. We'll be at the same school next year and I'm worried that she is going to wreck my chances of making new friends. Is there anything I can do to prevent this? Don't suggest that I go to a different school—I don't have a choice.

The answer to this question depends on what your relationship is like otherwise.

If you feel that you two get along OK except when it comes to your illness, it may be that she doesn't understand your condition and is making comments to try to draw attention to that. If you were diagnosed a long time ago, the information that she was given might have been too basic, or maybe she didn't understand it, or maybe no one explained anything. You could leave a pamphlet or some other description of your condition on her bed and see what happens.

Maybe she is scared about getting too close to you. If she is worried that you might get sicker, or even die, she may be trying to protect herself emotionally. If you think this is the case, it could help her to talk with the brothers or sisters of people with the same condition as yours.

If you don't get along, there are a few possibilities. One is that she is jealous of all the attention she thinks you get. Maybe she imagines you sitting at the hospital having intimate conversations with your mother. Maybe she feels that because of you your parents aren't there for her when she needs them. Try to create some opportunities for her to get more of their attention. Consider going for some of your appointments by yourself, if this is possible. Or if you need someone to drive you, suggest that your mother take you to your appointment and then go shopping or out for a coffee with your sister, and then pick you up at a pre-arranged time.

Does she think you are smarter or more likable or more artistic than she is? Maybe she's attacking what she sees as your only weakness. If your parents tend to compare the two of you, you could ask them to try to stop doing this. You can encourage her in her interests and show her that you think her strengths are important.

If you can't figure out a way to get her on your side, consider telling her that you don't understand why she says these things and what your concerns are. Tell her you expect her to refrain from making these comments at school. You might want to let her know that you think keeping things private is an important part of friendship and that you have never told people things about her that she wouldn't like to have spread around the school.

My parents came to Canada before I was born, and they haven't been back home to visit. Now that they both have Canadian citizenship and have saved some money, they would like to go back next summer. They just found out that my cousin's wedding is being delayed until then, and now they are worried about taking me. They say that if my cousin's fiancé's family meets me, they will not want their son to marry her, since I am a sign that there is "bad blood" in our family. I don't want to spoil anything, but I want to go on the trip, and I feel weird about my parents going without me and pretending that I don't exist.

This is a very tough situation. The idea that "bad blood" in families causes many chronic conditions exists in many places, including North America. Part of your feeling "weird" about not going is that it must seem to you that your parents are embarrassed by your condition. Their feelings about you going seem to be related to their worries about others' beliefs and do not mean that they are not proud of you and your accomplishments.

Do your relatives know about your condition? If your parents have told them, they could ask for advice. It may be that it wouldn't be an issue, or that there is some way around it. If they haven't told their own families, then this may be the real reason they don't want to take you.

Another place to get guidance would be within your community here. If there are people who have been supportive of your parents and accepting of you, they would be good people to consult with. A spiritual leader or someone with an important position within the community might have some insight into the situation.

If the issue really is the wedding, perhaps they could delay the trip until after it has taken place.

My brother hardly ever has friends over. He's always out, playing ball, going to other people's houses and stuff like that. He "accidentally" told me that this is because he doesn't know what people will think when they see me, and he is worried that they won't want to be friends anymore. This hurt my feelings but also made me feel sad for him. Is there anything I can do to help?

Your brother imagines people walking into your house and being confronted by a surprise—The Disabled Sister (or The Short Older Brother, or The Sibling Who Has Difficulty Communicating, or … whatever). He doesn't want to have to deal with their reaction, and he assumes that he hangs around with kids who would react badly.

Hopefully, he's wrong. If not, he needs a new bunch of friends. If his friends can't cope with your existence, they aren't going to be very understanding of other differences between people. However, he's going to have to figure this out on his own. It's unlikely that he will want to hear you telling him to dump his friends.

If it is the initial shock he's worried about, why can't he mention it in advance? If it isn't a big secret, then there won't be anything for people to be shocked by. You might even be able to go to his class or to an organization that he is a member of and talk to the people there.

If your brother were to talk to other kids who are in the same situation, this could really help. There may be a sibling support group for your particular disease or disability, or something more general offered through the hospital or clinic you go to. Ability Online (www.abilityonline.org) has chat rooms for siblings, and it might be easier to talk to other people online rather than in person. He can also read the stories of some siblings on a site called Band-Aides and Blackboards (see the Resources section at the back of this book).

> **I have mild cerebral palsy. My speech is somewhat slurred, and I have to speak slowly to be understood. I have a slight limp, and my coordination isn't very good. My parents have always acted as if there is nothing wrong with me. They get upset if anyone refers to me as disabled. I was nine before I even heard the term "cerebral palsy." My parents seem to think that I can do everything as well as the kids I know at school, and that I should never need extra help. Last week we had a big argument. They wanted me to try out for basketball. I know I can't make the team. I got mad and asked them why they pretend I'm the same as other kids. My dad said they knew if they had high expectations of me I would live up to them, and they don't want me sitting around whining about being disabled. I know I can do a lot, but I can't do everything.**

I'm sure your parents have your best interests at heart, but what they are doing is not helping you. You've probably wondered if they will love you if you can't do everything perfectly.

They need to understand that no one can do everything. Everyone operates with some kind of a disability, whether it be intellectual, physical or emotional.

If this is just a question of parenting styles and their approach to life, it will help to sit down and calmly explain your point of view. Do they think that people who wear glasses should be able to drive without them? Do they think that everyone can get an A in every class? I'm sure you can think of many more examples. Their assumption that you can do everything has probably led to you doing much more than if they had put as much effort into discouraging you. Let them know that you appreciate their support, that you like knowing they are behind you when you attempt something new, but that at the same time, like everyone else, you do have limits.

If your parents never accepted that they have a child who has more physical limitations than other children, you have a bigger problem on your hands, one that probably needs some outside help. If they can't see your side when you talk to them, this might be the case. You can suggest that it might be helpful to talk this out with a counselor. Your doctor can give you names of counselors in your area. You may have difficulty getting your parents to agree to this, as they sound like people who don't believe in getting help. If this is the case, be persistent, and consider enlisting your doctor's aid in convincing them.

If you don't feel up to fighting this out, but still want them to back off a bit, decide what things you want to concentrate on over the next year. Tell your parents that these areas are your priorities, and that you want to develop your capabilities in these things and not start new activities.

You might find it helpful to be in a support group with other teens with similar difficulties. Your local CP association should be able to help you find one (or you can encourage them to start a group).

Ever since I can remember, my uncle has been making little comments to me like "You know, you'll never get a man" and otherwise implying that my CF (cystic fibrosis) would stop me from being a "real" woman. It has always bothered me when he hugs me or touches me, but all my aunts and uncles hug me, so I couldn't really say anything. Lately he has been brushing against me, standing close behind me and commenting about my developing body. I told him he had to stop it because I didn't feel comfortable, but he said I was making it up. He said I was having fantasies about him because no boy my own age would be interested in me. He said that if I say anything to my parents he'll tell them that I have a crush on him! Now what do I do?

You have to tell one of your parents right away. If you don't, not only will your uncle's behavior continue but several studies show that this abuse escalates over time. Tell your parents everything he has said and done, including how he tried to get you to keep quiet. This will be hard, and there is the risk they won't believe you at first.

If you had just been imagining this, his response would likely have been to apologize for making you uncomfortable and to stop the behavior. The fact that he threatened you makes it quite clear that his actions were intentional.

This man has abused you in more than one way. Probably the most serious has been his comments. It is hard to feel good about yourself and your attractiveness when someone has been telling you for such a long time how unattractive you are. As you approached adolescence, you probably had concerns anyway about how your illness would affect your relationships. It would be difficult to resist believing him.

As sexual abusers often pick out children whom they see as being vulnerable, it stands to reason that kids who are different in any way, including having a chronic condition, are at increased risk for abuse. In fact, recent studies support this idea.

Remember, you are in no way responsible for what he has done. You are probably worried about the effect that telling your parents will have on your family. Any effect it has is his fault, not yours.

If you need to talk with someone about this before (or after) telling your parents, the hospital where you get treated for your CF probably has people who deal with sexual abuse. You could also talk to a guidance counselor or teacher whom you trust.

I have a facial deformity. The last time I went to the doctor he said that there is a new surgeon in town who does craniofacial surgery and suggested that I go to see him. I did, and he said that he could operate on me and that although the results wouldn't be perfect, there would be major improvement. My mother says I can't have the surgery. She says that I have adjusted well to my problem and that I have the face God meant me to have. I try to ignore people staring at me, but I still find it very difficult dealing with looking so different from everyone else. I'm almost 18 and no one has ever asked me out. How can I convince her that I should have the surgery?

It is very hard to argue with parents who feel that problems their child has been born with are there for a purpose—perhaps to punish the parents, or to make the child stronger. Rational arguments don't usually work in this case, because religious values come from belief and traditional wisdom rather than pure reason. Your mother's beliefs have helped her raise you and continue to affect your relationship with her.

It is unlikely to work, but I would start by explaining to your mother the impact that your appearance has on you. Try to point out that maybe whatever purpose it was meant to achieve has been fulfilled and that God may have sent this surgeon to reward you with a face that is easier for you to live with.

If these arguments don't work, talk to the surgeon and explain the situation. Ask him at what age he would do the surgery with your consent only. Legal age of consent varies from province to province and state to state, and you could check this out. I think there is a good chance that the surgeon would do the operation with your consent when you turn 18. Find out if there is a time limit—an age when the surgery will be most effective.

You've mentioned only your mother. If your father is living with you or is active in your life, maybe you can get him on your side and ask him to talk with your mother.

When you have the information from the surgeon, talk to both your parents. Don't make accusations like "You've ruined my life," and try to stay calm. Tell them you are considering having the surgery without their consent and see what the response is. Give them some time to think about it. They may just give in. Or they might say that they will kick you out or not pay for your university. You will have to make a decision that you can live with.

There is no question that it is difficult to live in a society where a large emphasis is placed on physical appearance.

There are probably people who have missed the chance to get to know you because you look different. There are also other factors that keep people apart, including everyone's insecurity.

Do not have unrealistic expectations of the effect this operation will have on your life. Try to talk with someone who has had similar surgery to discuss the effects. And before you have any operation, get as many details as you can about the possibility of a poor outcome both in how you look and your ability to function.

I have a hard time talking, and other people have difficulty understanding what I say. My parents almost always can figure out what I am saying, so they have been like translators for me for as long as I can remember. I just started at a regular high school this year, and I don't talk much. I would like to make more friends, and I don't want to involve my parents in helping me by translating for me. I don't think people will want to be friends with someone who brings his parents everywhere. What can I do to communicate without my parents? How will my parents feel about this?

I think your parents will be happy to see you growing up and becoming more independent. I'm sure that even though they will miss seeing you as much, once you are spending more time with friends they will be proud of your increasing ability to communicate.

You may want to explore alternative ways of communicating. In addition to typing things on your laptop computer and showing what you have typed (as you did to ask this question), you may want to look into text-to-voice software. All teens are comfortable with technology—unlike many of my generation—and will be interested by any device you may use.

Encourage people to interact with you by handing out cards that say something like "Hi, my name is _____ and I would like to talk to you. It may take some time for you to understand me, but I'd like to try." When you are talking, try to relax. If you are feeling really uptight, you will be harder to understand.

If you are not getting any speech therapy, consider going for some. The therapist may have suggestions about ways you can improve your communication.

Words are not the only way we communicate. You can indicate some of the things you want to say with hand gestures, facial expression, tone of voice, body language and volume. Make use of any of these that you can.

Always look at the person you are talking to. You may want to indicate to someone that he or she sit down if you are in a wheelchair, so that you are on the same level. (As well as improving communication, this can also change the power dynamics that exist when one person looks down at the other.)

Remember, when people seem to be frustrated when trying to understand you, they may be feeling that there is something wrong with them, not with you. I know when I have difficulty understanding someone, I feel it is me who is disabled in not being able to figure out what the person is saying.

I'm a 13 year old girl. When we got the puberty talk at school when I was 10, my mother told me that my vagina is very short and that I would have to get surgery and some medications at some point, but that it wasn't a big deal. When I went to see

my doctor recently, she told me that I am genetically male and that I have something called androgen insensitivity syndrome. I don't have a uterus and had surgery as a baby to take out testicles that were in my belly. She said that I don't have to have two X chromosomes to be a girl, and that I am likely to be tall and won't have acne (bonus!). I feel totally like a girl. I'm stunned!

I'm sure you are. This is a terrible way to find out something like this. The important thing for you to remember is that you are still the same person you were before. If you felt like a girl before, you are still a girl.

Many people assume that gender is a fairly straightforward thing—you're either male or female. In fact, it is a complex interaction of genes, hormones, fetal development and psychological factors. You are whatever gender you feel you are.

It is too bad your parents didn't tell you about this before. They probably had a hard time thinking of what to say to you. They may have felt they were giving you a "normal" childhood. I'm sure they felt it would be easier for you to understand when you were older. Maybe they were even planning to wait to tell you until you were an adult.

You are feeling upset and confused. We all develop a sense of who we are, what our bodies are about, as we grow up. When something changes, or when we discover something about ourselves that is different from what we had thought, it has a profound effect. Even very small differences can be disconcerting. Our self-identification as belonging to one gender or the other begins at a very young age. Therefore, information such as you have just received is a big shock.

I think you need some time to talk with someone about all this, to sort out your feelings and to be comfortable again with yourself. Although starting medication sometime in the next year or two might be a good idea, an operation at this time will just reinforce that there is something "wrong" with you, and this is not a helpful feeling at the best of times.

My mother understands some English, but she doesn't speak it. I translate for her when we go for appointments. I have been doing this since I was 10. I don't always translate everything. At first, I wanted to protect her from knowing how sick I was. She has lots of other things to worry about. Now, I am protecting myself too, because I know that she would want to keep me at home all the time and not let me have any freedom. But I am also feeling bad about lying to her, and I'm worried that I'll get caught, especially since her understanding of English is improving.

You'll be in a better position if you tell her, rather than being caught. I'd start by talking to her about how much you are able to do, and how your illness doesn't stop you from doing many activities. You can also point out any improvements there have been in your health to show that your activities have not been bad for your health.

Then explain to her that you are aware of many of her worries. Tell her you decided to protect her from knowing everything about your illness, but you feel it is time to tell her.

If she then says you have to stop doing things, you may want to point out to her that just as it wasn't right for you to protect her from knowledge of your condition, it isn't right for her to try to protect you from life. Go back to your previous conversation, and talk again of how much you can do, and how positive it makes you feel.

Secrets like this can lead to trouble. There is certainly nothing wrong with privacy. There will always be things you don't want to discuss with your mother. There may be times when you want to talk to your doctor without her there. But when you try to hide something like the nature of your illness, you have to constantly watch what you say. Dishonesty tends to creep into more of your relationship. In addition, you worry all the time that you will be found out. Perhaps you would have helped your mother learn more English if you hadn't been worried about protecting your secret.

I don't know what gets into me. I just get so mad and I get overwhelmed by it. I feel like I can't even see or hear when it is happening. I break things and yell, and the last time I hit my mother. Now she says I can't live at home anymore and is trying to find a place to send me to. She says that if I hit her again she'll call the police and I'll go to jail. I'm really scared about this. I don't want to go to jail or even move out but I don't feel like I can stop this. Things were so different before my head injury.

What probably "gets into" you is that parts of your brain that normally stop you from flying into a rage have been damaged and it is harder for you to control your behavior than it was before your injury. You may also be feeling pretty angry about all the ways your life has changed.

This doesn't mean that you are stuck with throwing things around and hitting people forever. I'm sure you realize that this is not a good thing to do, and right now the possible consequences are huge.

You need a plan to present to your mother. Coming up with this plan is something you can't do on your own. I suggest you get in touch with your doctor or clinic and make an appointment to discuss this. There may be a nurse-practitioner or social worker whom you feel you can talk with who can help you out. When you have come up with a plan, make sure you have it written down, with a copy for you and one for your mother.

Depending on what part of your brain has been affected, there might actually be some medication that would help. One drug that is used for this is called rispiradone. If your doctor thinks this might work for you, part of your plan will have to involve how you are going to remember to take it. If you need your mother to remind you to take it, part of the plan should be that you will take it when she reminds you, and not get annoyed with her for bugging you.

There might be occasions when you are more likely to have one of these outbursts. Maybe it is when you are really tired. It could be when you have a headache. It might be when there is a lot going on, like many people in the house, loud music playing, lots of chaos. Your plan should include how you are going to prevent these outbursts from happening. It might involve getting to bed at a certain time, taking something for a headache or lying down with your door shut when you have one. You may need to spend time alone by going for a walk or going to your room when things are crazy at home.

The clinic you go to might have a rehab therapist or behavior therapist who can help you with practical advice for your plan. If not, you might be able to see one privately if there is money available from an insurance settlement or health care insurance.

I think your plan should also include some ongoing counseling or therapy. You may be feeling angry or depressed about

the changes in your life. Maybe everything seems pretty hopeless at this point. A counselor can help you figure out who you
are and what you want to do with your life.

This plan will end up being a contract between you and
your mother that will guide the two of you. There will be things
for your mother to do (like making sure you get medication,
or maybe giving you a signal when she sees that things may be
going in the wrong direction). There will be things for you to
do. The plan should also say what happens if you don't follow
the plan. If people are telling you that you are having problems
with judgment, you should rely on the contract to tell you what
to do, rather than deciding that it doesn't apply in a situation.

You will still get mad (everyone does), but this should help
you control how you express it and hopefully allow you to stay
at home.

**I need help getting dressed in the morning. To
make things easier, and to save time, my mother
buys me loose clothes, sometimes two or three
sizes too big. Clothes are pretty important
where I go to school and I'd like to be dressed
more fashionably. How can I convince her?**

To start with, have you talked with her about this? Most teenagers buy their own clothes, either with their mothers or with
friends.

Explain to your mother how you feel. Don't be surprised
if she tells you that what you wear isn't important, it's who you
are inside. Although this is true (really), it isn't helpful information. Many teens judge others by what they wear. In addition, what you wear influences how you feel. Tell her that if you
feel dowdy (I know no one uses that word anymore, but I like

it) wearing a tent instead of a sweater, you are going to feel that no one will want to talk with you and you will send this feeling out into the world.

Present your mother with a proposal. If there is a time of year when she buys most of your clothes, ask for control of part of the budget (at least 25%, and make sure she's responsible for the things that don't matter as much to you). Plan some of your purchases ahead of time, and decide what is the most you can spend on various types of clothes. Don't buy anything that doesn't go with the rest of your clothes (you may want to plan around a color scheme). Assume that you will make a few mistakes and don't get too upset by them.

There are some clothes that you shouldn't buy without trying on, unless the store has a good return policy and you know it won't be too much hassle to get back to exchange things. You will need to allow plenty of time for trying things on. Make sure you and your mother have something to eat before you go out so you don't get too grumpy.

There are clothes that are fashionably baggy. Consider including some in your wardrobe. In all clothes, look for things that might make them easier to put on, such as a large neck or arm holes.

Allow for the extra time it will take to get ready in the morning. You may have to get up earlier. Don't skip breakfast to gain a few minutes. You need your energy to get through a morning at school. Make sure you stick with your plan, so that when it is time to buy more clothes, your mother can't tell you that you don't have the time to dress the way you want.

Whenever I meet a girl in a wheelchair who is around my age, my mother talks about how nice she is, how cute she is, how smart she is

and encourages me to get to know her better. It doesn't seem to matter what she is actually like. Does she think a guy in a chair is only interested in a girl in one? How can I get her off my back?

Your mother is probably afraid that no one will be interested in a relationship with you. She probably feels that someone who is also in a wheelchair will understand your situation better and will be attracted to you.

I am sure that she doesn't realize how demeaning this is to you (and to these girls, who are seen as suitable only because they share a diagnosis with you).

Your mother may be concerned that she hasn't seen you taking an interest in girls and feels that this would be a safe and easy place for you to start. She may be thinking that you are gay and is pushing these girls on you to prove to herself that you aren't.

Maybe she feels that a friendship or relationship based on having something in common with the other person will be a strong and lasting one.

The easiest way to find out is to ask her why she is doing this. Try not to confront her or she will just get defensive. Explain to her that you want to choose whom you relate to, and that diagnosis is not your main criteria in a relationship. Let her know you won't discriminate against people just because they have the same condition as you, but at the same time, it isn't the main thing you are looking for.

All mothers do this to their kids. They pick out people who are acceptable to them and promote them to their teens. When asked, they usually deny they are doing this, saying, "I just mentioned that I thought she was a nice girl. I'm entitled to my opinion."

The good thing about this is that your mother is seeing you as someone who is growing up. She is expressing her assumption that you will be getting involved with people, which is much better than having a parent who thinks you shouldn't be moving out into the world.

I was in the hospital for over a month just after I was diagnosed. The day I came home, my dad moved out. I've heard my mother talking to friends about how stressful my illness has been for her, and I'm worried that it caused my parents to break up. I know if I asked my mother about it, she would say it wasn't my fault, but I'm not sure that I can trust her to tell the truth.

There is no doubt that the stress of a child's illness is hard on parents, and shaky relationships may break down in the face of this stress. However, no marriage breaks up in a month. Your parents must have been having problems for a long time before your father left. Sometimes, one person has been unhappy in a marriage without talking about it, so it seems sudden to the other person. If things had been working as they should, they would have been communicating all along and would have tried to work through the problems before.

Just because your parents weren't fighting before you got sick doesn't mean things were going well. They may have drifted so far apart that they didn't care enough to get angry.

What about the timing of all this? It may be that your illness was one last stress on a relationship that was breaking up anyway, the straw that broke the camel's back. Or your mother may have decided to put up with the relationship until you got sick, but then realized that if she couldn't have a supportive partner, it would be better to have none.

This was an awful time for your father to leave. Maybe he was waiting to make sure you would be all right. Maybe he was so angry with your mother (or she with him) that he didn't stop to think about the effect on you.

Yes, it is hard on parents to have a child who is ill. Worrying constantly (and they do) can make them grumpy and short with each other. Especially around the time of diagnosis, their child needs a lot more attention, and that may mean the parents have little time or energy to spend on their own relationship. This added stress can be hard on a marriage that is already in trouble, but it does not mean the added stress causes the marriage to break up.

You have probably also worried about whether your father still loves you, or whether your illness makes you unlovable in some way. Neither is true. Your father is surely distressed about your condition. Maybe he finds it hard to see you if you are in pain. But he still loves you.

Your worries about this have probably affected your mood and your ability to deal with your illness. Try to understand that you have not caused your parents to split up. Consider talking to your mother about how you have been feeling. She may be thinking that your silence on the subject of the breakup is because you blame her for it.

I'm a 13-year-old guy who needs help with getting undressed, bathing and getting ready for bed at night. My parents both help me, more often my mother. If my parents go out, my mother gets my aunt or a neighbor to help me. I am starting to feel pretty embarrassed about

it. I guess I can stand my mother doing it, although I'm not thrilled about it, but I really don't want these other women seeing me with no clothes on. They'd probably say they don't even notice, but to me, that makes it worse. It means that I'm just like a little kid to them, instead of someone who is almost a man.

Kids grow up so gradually that parents sometimes don't notice how grown up their kids are unless it is pointed out to them. Your mother has been doing the same routine for so long that it is probably pretty automatic. She may enjoy interacting with you at this time and not pay much attention to your body, or maybe she thinks about other things entirely.

I'm sure part of the reason you haven't talked with her yet is that you don't want her to stop going out so that she can be home to get you ready. And you may feel it would be too much of a burden for your father to do more of your care. They are unlikely to know how you feel unless you talk to them.

If you and your father can talk to each other, why not approach him first? Ask him if he could help you more and explain why. Let him know that you understand he can't do it all the time, but that you would appreciate it if he could increase the frequency of helping you.

When your parents go out, would it be possible for you to stay up until they get home? Or, if you aren't having friends over, maybe you could get ready early, before they go out. Maybe they could get a volunteer from an organization they belong to, or pay someone to stop in and help you.

Is there a possibility that you will be able to learn to do these things independently? There may be some styles of clothing that would be easier to change in and out of. If you go to a clinic, ask to talk to an occupational therapist, who may be able to help you learn to transfer in and out of the shower or bathtub, get ready for bed and get dressed in the morning.

If it is not going to be possible for you to do these things unassisted, you and your family need to start thinking about long-term solutions to this problem. Your mother is not always going to be there to do these things for you. Part of being an adult involves managing without your mother's help, at least some of the time. Ask your parents for some time when you can sit down and talk about what's bothering you.

My mother and I were having a fight last week about my curfew (too early) when she said, "It's bad enough that I gave you this disease. I'm not going to let you get into unsafe situations." I asked her what she meant, but she wouldn't answer. My parents have always told me that my illness wasn't my fault, that I am not responsible for it. Is she saying that she is?

Parents often feel their children's problems are their fault, and this is especially true of parents who have children with disabilities or illnesses.

If you were born with your condition, your mother probably feels that she either gave it to you by passing on the gene that caused it, or by not taking care of herself well enough when she was pregnant or by not eating the right things.

As you were growing up, she may have hidden these feelings from herself by throwing herself into your care. She could keep herself so busy worrying about you, taking you to appointments and providing for your needs that she wouldn't have time to think about all of this.

Now, as you are getting older and are taking more responsibility for yourself, she may be flooded with feelings of guilt.

Consider talking with her about this. Tell her that you feel she needs to work through her feelings about this, because not only do they make her unhappy but she is using them to limit your activities. Let her know that you don't want her to have to feel guilty in five years for having overprotected you as a teenager. It may be that she will not let you talk with her about this at all, or she may not be able to respond.

Try not to complicate matters further by feeling guilty about how guilty she feels about your condition. She can change how she is feeling, and how she has chosen to feel is in no way your fault.

Continue to press for independence. Find ways of expressing your individuality—through the way you dress, your hairstyle, the music you listen to, the friends you choose. You need to be looking after your personal growth at a time when her guilt prevents her from doing so.

I must be the first teen ever to complain about this. I don't have any chores to do at home. My brother and sister both have things they have to do. They each have two "everyday" jobs—making up their beds and one other thing like washing the dishes. Then they have a "weekend" job like washing the kitchen floor or cleaning the bathroom. They both feel resentful that I don't help out. I feel useless.

You are right—it isn't a usual complaint, but it is a valid one. Chores play an important role as we grow up. When you perform a job, you feel like a contributing member of your family.

Household tasks also give you experience so that when you go out on your own, you will know how to do some basic things.

The kinds of messages that you get when you are denied an active place in the maintenance of your family are that you are not competent to do the jobs and would end up being a burden, and that you do not need independence skills, because you will never be independent.

I am not saying these are the messages your parents want you to get. They probably think they are sparing you in some way. But if you aren't allowed to participate as a full family member, you aren't going to feel competent. You will have a sense of being someone who is taken care of, rather than being someone who is in control of his or her life. You will have to live with the resentment of your siblings, when you'd be better off to have them as allies.

Start by tackling some jobs when your parents aren't home. Tell your brother and sister that you want to start doing stuff. Pick a job and get competent. You may have to adjust the job to your own abilities. If you get tired easily, take breaks. Find ways to make the job less tiring (there's no rule that says you can't vacuum sitting on the floor). When you feel good about it, let your parents know that this will be your job for the next while. Make sure they know this was your idea. Tell them why it is important to you.

They may be pleased. But they may be upset because they are used to doing everything for you. It may make one of them feel useless to think that one day you won't need them to take care of you. You can remind them that you will always need them to love you.

Once the initial thrill wears off, there will be days when you would rather be doing something else. You'll need to remind yourself of why this task is important. In the long run, you will feel better about yourself and your capabilities. And when you do move out, you'll know how to keep your place clean.

Last week when I went to the clinic, my mother asked to speak with the doctor alone. After, I asked her what she had talked with him about and she said it wasn't my concern. But he's my doctor, so she must have been talking about me. Is she allowed to do this?

He is your doctor, but what they were discussing may not have related directly to you.

Maybe your mother has been feeling depressed or upset and wanted some advice about whom she could speak with. Although you may have noticed how she was feeling, she still doesn't have to discuss it in front of you. It may not even have a direct relationship to your condition. Believe it or not, you aren't the sole focus of your parents' lives!

There may have been something about your behavior that has been bothering your mother. She might not have wanted to discuss it with you until she had a chance to talk with someone else. If your doctor had felt it was something to worry about, he probably would have suggested talking with the two of you that day. He might have told her that it is normal behavior for a teen and she doesn't need to worry about it.

There may be a financial problem related to your condition that your mother wanted to discuss. She may have wanted to talk about it privately so you wouldn't have to worry about it. Doctors can often give advice about funding agencies and other options.

Your parents need to be able to get support. They have rights to privacy, just as you do. If you have questions that you don't want to ask in front of your mother or something you want to talk about, you can ask to talk to the doctor by yourself, and you don't have to tell your mother what it is about, any more than she has to tell you. Next time you see your doctor, you can explain that you were worried about what they were discussing, and clarify that you don't want him talking about what you have said to him without your permission.

My parents recently told me that I am HIV positive. I had heart surgery in another country when I was born and had a lot of blood transfusions, but I assumed that I was negative because they hadn't told me otherwise. I feel pretty mad about this (I could have given it to someone), but now I'm even more upset because they are saying I shouldn't talk to anyone about it, not even our family. When are they going to tell my relatives—when I'm dead?

Having a big secret in a family can lead to real problems. For one thing, in your case, the message you get is that being HIV positive is so horrible that no one else can know about it. You may even be feeling that you are a bad person to have acquired the virus. A secret reinforces the idea that you can trust and rely on only the people in your immediate family, which isolates you from many sources of support.

When your parents found out that you were HIV positive, they probably had a number of reasons for not telling you. They may have thought they were sparing you the pain of finding out. They may have wanted to find out more about HIV before telling you. They may have even been advised by your doctor not to tell you (is there a rule that says doctors can't do stupid things sometimes?).

It is obviously important to you not to keep this a secret. Your parents need to know that this is your information, and it is up to you to decide whom to tell.

Think about which of your relatives are likely to be supportive and tell them first. Have all the information you need to answer their questions. You may even want to give them some pamphlets from your local AIDS organization. Their loving response will help your parents cope with the "secret" being revealed.

It may be that not all your relatives will react in a positive manner. Some may not understand that they and their children are safe and cannot get the virus from being around you, kissing you or eating off the same dishes. You need to educate yourself about HIV and then you can help other people understand it better.

By the way, don't assume that you are going to die from this condition. You have lived this long with it, and it sounds as though you are doing pretty well. If you are on medications, taking them at the right time and not missing doses will greatly increase your chance of living with HIV, rather than dying from AIDS.

It is unlikely that I will ever be able to move out of my parents' house. So why do people at the clinic keep talking to me about independence? Are they trying to make me feel unhappy with my family? My family is the best support anyone could ever have.

Independence means learning to rely on yourself for as much as you can, and to take responsibility for your thoughts and actions. No one is totally independent. Unless you lived on an island all by yourself, grew or caught your food and made your clothes, you would be dependent on others for some of the basics of daily life. And even on the island, you'd be dependent on the earth and what it can give you. Independence also means having a world that goes beyond your family. But this can be achieved while living with your parents.

An important part of being a teen is learning what you can do for yourself and figuring out how you feel about world issues. It means developing a sense of ideals that in some way define who you are and what you believe in.

Independence and separation from parents are often linked. Part of independence is having a more adult relationship with your parents. It can be harder to achieve this when you don't have a chance to be away from them. But it can be done.

Start to take responsibility for your body. You can be the one to decide what to wear, when to bathe or wash your hair and what hairstyle to have. You can remember to take your medication. Even if you need help with all these things, you can still make decisions about them. You may be able to do more of your care than you think. If you need injections, maybe you can learn how to do this. If you need catheterization, perhaps you can learn how. If that isn't possible, maybe you can get everything ready and be in charge of when it is going to happen.

Make sure you have jobs around the house. These can be suited to what you can do. If you are physically unable to clean things, maybe you can do menu planning or work on the shopping list. Maybe you can sort the clothes for the laundry.

Find out about various social issues and take a stand on them. You may want to change your mind as you learn more, but don't be afraid to have an opinion. Think about religion. Find out what your family and friends really believe. You may want to attend religious services with friends of different faiths, not to change what you believe but to help you understand different ways of believing.

Plan your own study schedule. Decide which courses are a priority for you and put extra work into them.

Develop a hobby or an interest in something. Find out if you can get together with other people interested in the same thing, either in person or online.

Make sure you understand what your condition is really all about. Consider helping someone who has been more recently diagnosed who could use some support.

Think about who you are romantically interested in (if you aren't now, don't worry, this will come at some point). Notice if you are attracted to certain types of people. You will want to find ways of getting to know these people and making friends with them.

Explore your sexuality. When you have sexual feelings, don't push them away. Fantasize about what you like. Read the chapter in this book about sex (Chapter 6).

You don't have to go out tomorrow and do all these things. Pick something and work on it for a while. When it becomes routine, add something else in.

Remember, it is up to you to decide what independence means for you.

My parents have always fought for my independence. I have been in integrated classes, and when I finished high school I got job training and I have a job. I plan to move out soon, and I can't believe their reaction. They didn't react like this when my older brother moved out, or when my sister got married, so it can't be because I am a girl. It must be because of my condition. They don't seem to be able to let me go.

Your assumption may not be totally correct.

It sounds as though you are the youngest in your family. It can be difficult for parents to see their last child leave. It changes who they are (parents with kids at home) and will mean doing some thinking about their own goals and their future.

Because you are the youngest, your parents may see you as the "baby" of the family. They may be in the habit of seeing you as less competent than your older siblings because of this.

Your parents may also have some concerns about unmarried girls moving out. They may have a double standard, where it is all right for your brother to be living away from home but it's not for you. They may think you are moving out so that you can have sex, and they may be scared about that.

Your condition may also play a part in this. They may see you as needing more help, as being vulnerable to many of the challenges of living on your own. If you have been limited in your opportunities to get out and socialize, they may worry that you don't have the skills to handle yourself in social situations.

They are probably worried that moving out will cause unhappiness.

It would be helpful for you and your parents to sit down with someone (maybe a social worker from the clinic where you go, or someone from an advocacy organization) and talk this out. Your parents need some help in accepting the fact that you are ready to move out. Reassure them that you have thought through financial and safety issues. Let them know you are not deserting them, but set out some rules, such as no dropping by without calling first.

In a way, your parents are going through a developmental stage. Until now, their job has been to help you get through your developmental stages in a positive way. Now the roles have switched, and you need to help them move on.

I am 13 and my mother still catheterizes me. I tried to learn how a couple of years ago, but I kept dropping things and I was slow. It was faster for her to do it. I would like to try to learn again, but I don't want to make life more difficult for her. She already gives me more of her time than my brothers and sisters get.

Even if it takes you a while, in the end this is going to save your mother time. Just as you sometimes have to spend money to make money, sometimes you have to use time to save time.

You are getting to an age where being able to take care of your body functions is important. If you are female, you will need to learn to put on a menstrual pad or insert a tampon when you get your period, and learning to catheterize yourself is an important first stage in taking on responsibility for your body.

Catheterizing is a private thing. Whether you are male or female, you are not going to want other people of either sex touching your genitals as if this was any other part of your body. Not everybody can catheterize themselves (you have to be able to use your arms and hands), but if you have the capability, you should learn how.

Time passes quickly, and it may seem to your mother that your attempt to learn was recent, and not a couple of years ago.

Let her know that it is time for you to start learning again. If she says it will be too much work, point out that she didn't keep your siblings in diapers forever just because toilet training was work.

If there is a time when things aren't as rushed (maybe bedtime), this would be a good time to practice. You may be able to get lessons at the clinic where you go (after all, someone taught your mother). When you have gained confidence, you can take over the other times.

If you and your mother use these times to talk now, you may want to find an opportunity to have 5 or 10 minutes to talk every day when she no longer has to help you.

My father doesn't spend much time with me. When we do go out, I like it. He and I do different things than I do with my mother. He lets me take more risks. Is there anything I can do to have more time with him?

Many kids with disabilities or illnesses say that their fathers are not as protective as their mothers. This isn't surprising. It is much more common for mothers to be home full time with their children, and they get into the routine of taking care of them. It can be harder for them to let go.

All families these days find there just isn't enough time. Your father may want to spend more time with you but think he doesn't have the time.

Is there a job your father normally does that you could take over? If you could do it during the week, it might free up some time for you on the weekend.

Are you and your father putting off spending time together until you have a large chunk of free time, like a whole afternoon? If you are, then you may be waiting forever. What about just seeing if he wants to go out for half an hour? You could go out for a walk or a cup of coffee. If you get into the habit of doing this regularly, it may fill the same need. And if a big block of time becomes available, he is more likely to think of spending it with you if he is in the habit of going out with you for shorter times.

Does your father have a hobby that you could get interested in? If he spends time on it every week, he may be happy to share this time with you.

Does your father know that you would like to be with him more? Maybe he thinks your mother does such a good job of taking care of you that there is nothing left for him to do. Make sure you tell him you are trying to think of ways that the two of you could be together more.

I live with my grandmother, and I appreciate her taking me in and giving me so much love. But we are having a big problem around my getting a summer job. I want one. I need the experience and I'd like to have the extra money. I'd also like to give her some money, because I know how hard it is for her sometimes to support both of us. She says that if I get a job, people will think she can't take care of me. She thinks that people back home will hear about it and think I shouldn't live with her anymore.

First, you have to figure out if she is worried about what other people will think or if she also has these same concerns. Does she think that you want a job because you think she doesn't support you well enough? Does she see this whole thing as a rejection of what she has given you?

If these are her concerns, then you need to deal with them. Make sure she knows how much you appreciate what she has done for you. Point out that she has helped you become a strong, independent person who will be able to support herself in a few years. Let her know that you still need her.

If she is truly concerned about her friends both here and at home, there may be some ways to get around it.

You might think that getting a job you can do online would solve this issue, but the social aspects of work are important. I would suggest you do online work only as a last resort.

If you are likely to get a job that her friends won't find out about, she could just say that you are going to summer school or something similar. They don't have to know what you are doing. However, she may want to let her friends know that you are doing so well now that she hardly thinks of you as having a problem. She can tell them how much you are able to do, and that she thinks you are even ready to learn to accept some responsibility and get a summer job. She can talk about it in terms of what you will be learning, rather than what you will be earning.

2

Doctors and Medical Issues

DOCTORS AND OTHER HEALTH CARE PROVIDERS have an influence on your life that may be greater than any adults other than your parents. You may feel that too much of your time is taken up by them, that they have too much say about what happens to you, that your parents listen to them too much. You may like your doctor; you may hate her. You may feel that your nurse-practitioner isn't interested in you as a person, or that he is nosy and interested in things that are none of his business.

Whatever you can do to improve your relationship with your health care team will help improve the quality of your life.

This chapter addresses questions about how to deal with doctors, hospitals and health care workers and answers some specific medical questions.

How can I talk to my doctor about some things that are really bothering me? He's a really nice guy but he's always in a hurry and my parents are usually in the room. Most of the time I want them there, but this stuff is too personal.

Doctors can get very busy, but almost all of them are willing to take time to listen to you. The problem is that many doctors aren't very good at communicating this and unconsciously use all kinds of non-verbal cues (glancing at a watch, standing up while talking instead of sitting down, etc.) that show that we are in a hurry. Have you tried just asking your doctor if you can talk to him alone? You might want to tell your parents first and reassure them that you want them there for most of the appointment. If your doctor doesn't have the time, or if he says he does but is obviously distracted, ask if you can make an appointment to talk to him for 15 minutes or half an hour.

If you go to a clinic, there might be a nurse-practitioner you could talk with—this is a big part of her job. When you have questions she can't answer, she will talk with the doctor or other members of the team to seek advice.

What can you do if your doctor is unwilling to talk with you alone, your parents cannot help you convince him to change his mind and there is no nurse to speak with?

If this doctor is a specialist in your condition, you probably have a family doctor whom you see for other problems. Approach her with your questions. She might not be able to answer them immediately, but she should be able to talk with the specialist herself to get the answers for you.

If the questions you have don't directly relate to your condition, a health care practitioner in a different field might be able to help you.

Over the long term, you will have to decide whether you want a doctor who doesn't talk to you. You might consider switching to someone who is willing to recognize you as a person with a right to privacy and dignity.

I'm new to this being sick thing, and it is all very confusing. Everybody at the hospital seems to have a different title—there seem to be about six levels of doctors. Can you explain who all these people are?

Doctors go through a number of stages of education and training, and each of these has a name. It used to be easy to figure out who everyone was because they wore different uniforms. Now, you can't tell who someone is by his or her clothes, but all doctors and other staff in hospitals are supposed to wear name tags that say who they are and where they are in their training. If you know the code (explained below), you can tell what level they are at. Some hospitals have few of these doctors-in-training, but if there are enough of them to confuse you, your hospital probably has full training programs in a number of fields.

A **medical student** is in a three- or four-year program to learn to be a doctor. Most have a university degree already. Their name tag may say what year they are in. The years are school years, not calendar years, so in April a fourth-year student is going to be a doctor in a couple of months. In England and some places in Canada, medical students in the last part of their training are called **clinical clerks**, or just **clerks**, so don't get worried if someone says a clerk is going to examine you. A clerk can do some things without direct supervision but shouldn't be performing complicated procedures without being accompanied by a doctor. A medical student should never introduce himself or herself as "Doctor So and So."

After graduating from medical school, doctors must have further training—like an apprenticeship. A one-year **internship** is required in many places before a doctor can get a license. If someone has a name tag that identifies him as a **rotating intern**, this does not mean that he spins around (although he might feel as though he does). This intern rotates through several different specialties during the year.

To be a specialist or a family doctor (as opposed to a general practitioner), a doctor must do a **residency**. Residents rotate through different areas within their specialty. Different specialties have differing lengths of training, the shortest being two years for family practice. A resident's name tag may tell you what year of training she is in.

You may hear interns and residents referred to as **house staff** or **house officers**. This comes from the days when they literally lived "in house"—at the hospital. Interns and residents still stay overnight every few nights, which is why they sometimes look so rotten in the morning.

Fellows spend between one and three years learning a specialty within a specialty. They have already been residents and provide quite a bit of care without direct supervision. However, there is always a **staff doctor** responsible for your care. This person has finished all of his training and has taken special exams.

It may seem to you that all of these trainees are practicing on you, and that you could get better care if you had one or two doctors taking care of you, instead of a herd. But having trainees in a hospital keeps the quality of care high. Staff doctors have to be knowledgeable about new ideas in their field to stay ahead of the house staff. And it means that more people are thinking about you and your condition.

There are many other health care workers in any hospital. As with doctors, uniforms are not an easy way for them to be identified. Most hospitals do not require nurses to wear caps. There may be several levels of nurses, with **nurse's aides**, **registered nursing assistants** (called **licensed practical nurses** in some places), **registered nurses**, **nurse-clinicians**, **nurse-specialists and nurse-practitioners** all working together. Their responsibilities vary widely from hospital to hospital, so ask nurses at the various levels what they do. You may also be cared for by physical therapists (also called physiotherapists), occupational therapists, psychologists, social workers and

Child and Youth Councilors. If they don't explain who they are and what they will do with you, ask them. The other workers you will see frequently will usually be involved in a specific task—drawing blood, taking an X-ray, transporting you from place to place—so it is easier to figure out what they do.

Not only will you sort people out by rank, you will also get to know many of them and will come into contact with them when you come to outpatient appointments. The resident who examines you today may be the staff doctor in charge of your care in four years.

I'm a 14-year-old paraplegic. I'm recovering from a pressure sore on my bum (an embarrassing location) and am anxious to prevent another one, having spent a boring two months in bed on my belly. My doctor just tells me to be more careful. I don't find this very helpful! What can I do so that this doesn't happen again?

I can see why you are frustrated by your doctor's advice. For one thing, it implies that you were being careless before and that you know how to prevent pressure sores. If this is your first one, she might have assumed that you knew how to prevent them. She hasn't considered that, now that you're 14 years old, there are several factors that might have led to this sore that didn't exist before.

You are probably taking more responsibility for your own care now and are having to learn to do a lot of new things. Some things might have been so automatic to your care-giver that he or she has forgotten to mention them to you. Your skin should be clean and dry as much as possible. If you are getting sweaty playing sports or just in the mad dash between classes, you need to find the time to get dried off during the day.

You are starting to grow quickly and might be outgrowing your wheelchair or your clothes. Pressure sores form when soft tissues such as muscle and skin are pressed between a bone and another object, which lessens the flow of blood to these tissues. Friction can also lead to pressure sores. Clothes that are too tight or a wheelchair that rubs may be the culprit.

As school gets harder and classes get longer, you may be sitting still for too long. You should be shifting your position every 15 minutes. If you feel this will make you stick out in class, look around you. None of your classmates are sitting perfectly still throughout class.

Are you getting thin as you get taller? Fat tissue cushions you and helps prevent pressure sores. Make sure you are getting enough to eat and that you are not skipping meals in your rush to get from one activity to another. Your diet should contain a good balance of food groups. Junk food is an essential emotional nutrient in adolescence, but don't overdo it. Excess weight can also lead to pressure sores.

If you can identify one or more of these as the cause of the sore, let your doctor know. Mention that the next time she sees a teen with a pressure sore, it would be helpful if she could be more specific. Tell her that you did feel you were being careful, but that you needed more information. You could also suggest to your doctor that if your hospital has a nurse who is a specialist in wound care or pressure sores, a referral would be helpful for you and other people in your predicament.

The nurse-practitioner at my doctor's office is pretty good at explaining things and has given me some pamphlets about my illness. I'd really like to have more information but when I went to the library at the hospital, everything was written for doctors and I couldn't really understand it. Where else can I find out stuff?

Depending on your illness, there might be a book written about it. You could check at the public library.

The Internet is often the easiest way to get information. Many adults start with Wikipedia, which generally gets corrected quickly when it presents misinformation. The problem with the Internet is that anyone can write and post anything, so you have to try to figure out if what you are reading can be trusted. In general, a site that is selling a treatment is not as trustworthy as one that isn't. Some of these are pretty obvious, but others don't make it clear that they are promoting a particular drug or remedy.

When doing a search on Google or another search engine, narrow things down by using several words in the search. If the name of your illness has more than one word, put the name in quotation marks. Think about including the word "adolescent" or "teen" in the search, so you don't get stuff that may not be as relevant to you.

Once you have gotten more information, you can go back to your nurse-practitioner with what you have learned and see if it matches with what she knows. She might have newer information, or be able to help clarify some of what you have learned.

There are numerous sites for young people with disabilities, including Ability Online, TeensHealth, and Band-Aides and Blackboards. You can read other people's stories, get information about your condition and maybe even link up with others in the same boat as you.

Many people get up-to-date information and links to new research through Twitter. You can get deluged with information this way, and may have to wade through multiple re-tweets, but you soon learn to be discerning about what links may be helpful or interesting to you. Twitter can be a way to connect with people who have similar views as you, or who share a common cause or condition.

When I go to a new clinic or see a new resident or medical student, they ask a lot of questions that I can't remember the answers to. Why can't they just read my chart? And if I can't get them to read it, then what can I do to remember this stuff?

There are many reasons for doctors to ask all these questions. One is that your chart might be very long and not something that they can easily skim. Also, things that aren't quite right can creep into a chart, so it is good to get the information directly from a patient. We teach medical students to "take a history" from the beginning.

There are two things that might help you. At my hospital, we encourage young people to learn a three-sentence summary, to be able to tell a new health care provider the most important things about your condition and treatment in three to four sentences. Medical students do this all the time. They meet you and ask you questions, then they "present" to the doctor in charge. A student might say something like, "Jose is a 16-year-old who had a kidney transplant for FSGS after being on dialysis for two years. He is six months post-transplant and his mother was his donor. He is on FK, MMF, prednisone, amlodipine, calcium and vitamin D. He has no new issues today." These are the type of things that you know about your condition or could memorize. If you can present yourself to a new health care practitioner in this way, they are unlikely to interrupt you and will feel confident that you are a knowledgeable patient who should be listened to.

For more detail, and to be used in emergencies when you can't speak or are too stressed to remember your information, carry a wallet-sized card stating your important health details. It is called MyHealth Passport and is created by a program that is available for free at www.sickkids.ca/myhealthpassport. You can chose from about 50 templates (or if your condition or group of conditions isn't listed, use the Generic Passport template), put in a very small amount of non-identifying data that will be saved in the system, and then fill in the other fields. Lots just require checkboxes. It is useful to do this with a nurse or doctor who is familiar with your details. When you are done, you can e-mail it to yourself and also print it. Cut along the lines, fold and then pop it into your wallet. The whole process takes most people fewer than 15 minutes. All your information is wiped from the system afterward, so you don't have to worry about your details being read by someone else.

I know that at age 16 I should be able to cope better with hospitalizations, but I can't! I hate sitting around all day, waiting for things to happen. I hate being in a room with babies and toddlers. I can't stand nighttimes—the noise, the loneliness, the uncomfortable beds. Is there any way I can adjust to this?

If by "adjust" you mean meekly accept it all, no. Even if you could, it would just make you a passive person who doesn't take control.

When you are well enough to be up and around, figure out a daily schedule. Write in when the doctors go on rounds. (You'll probably have to block off at least an hour, maybe more. Even though you see them for only a few minutes, they will usually see new patients first and you'll be waiting around for them to come.) Mark down the times that meals are served. Every morning, ask your nurse when she will need you around for medications or treatments. If there is a teacher at your hospital, reserve a block of time for him. The rest of the time is yours, as long as your nurse knows where to find you. What can you do in a hospital? If you are in a children's hospital, there may be a teen lounge where you can hang out, play video games or pinball, and get to know other teens in the hospital. If there is only one play area for all ages, see if you can find other patients your age and take over a corner of it. Take a book to the cafeteria or the main waiting area. If the weather is nice, go outside. In some hospitals, you may have to be accompanied by a nurse or volunteer. Usually the ones who smoke are pleased to get outside.

If you have to stay in your room, and you don't want to risk having a computer or game console from home being stolen, find out if there are computers on carts that can be loaned out to patients. If your hospital has a Child Life department, it is probably in charge of this.

Keep a bag packed with projects that can be done in the hospital. Crossword puzzles, hand-held video games, sewing, knitting (lots of guys knit, so this hobby isn't limited to just one gender) or a sketch pad and colored pencils are some things that can be included.

When you are admitted, let the people on the ward know that you understand it can be difficult for them to give you the roommate of your choice, but that if possible you prefer not to be with little kids. If you are in a general hospital, you may want to consider asking to be on an adult ward, but don't rush into this—speaking from personal experience, they tend to be very boring and you may not be any happier with a 90-year-old than a 9-month-old.

Try to space out your visitors so that everybody doesn't come on the same day. Invite friends to come and do homework or watch a video with you. They may be scared to come because they don't know what they'll do. If you have a friend you'd like to see who hasn't come to the hospital before, ask a friend who does visit to bring him or her.

If you have Internet access, stay in touch with your friends through your favorite social networking site. This is a good time to expand your network, perhaps with an already established group for people with your condition.

If your diet isn't restricted, see if family members and friends can bring real food. Maybe some friends could bring a pizza. Even if you have dietary restrictions, there are often things people can bring that you are allowed to eat.

Nighttime is the worst, there's no question about it. There isn't much you can do about the noise. If you still get woken up by the sound of the alarm on your IV (lots of teens tell me they can sleep through it), consider buying a pocket-sized timer and lending it to your nurse. If she expects your IV to run for two hours before it needs to be refilled, ask her to set it for an hour and 55 minutes, so that she can fill up the IV before the machine beeps. When you are first admitted, you will probably need to have your vital signs measured in the middle of the night. As you feel better, this might not be needed, but doctors often forget to change the orders. When they are on rounds, ask them if you still need to be woken up in the middle of the night for this.

If people are talking loudly at the nursing station, you can let them know by saying something about overhearing their conversation like "I was so interested to hear about your divorce. I can't believe that your husband really left you for an 18-year-old" or "I was amazed to hear that you don't like Dr. So and So. I'll ask him to be nicer to you." If you don't overhear what they are saying, you can wander out in the hall acting dazed and say, "Is it morning? It sounded like there were a whole bunch of people out here."

I think they cover hospital pillows with recycled yogurt containers. They are hard and crackle every time you move. Always bring your own pillow to the hospital. Bring your own pillowcases too, not just because they may be softer but to identify your pillow. Hospitals are notorious for terrible temperature control, and when you are sick you may feel colder than the people around you. Consider bringing a washable comforter. They are warmer than hospital blankets and have a cozier feel.

If you have a good luck charm, always take it with you. If it is something small, make or buy a bag for it so that it won't get lost.

No one is too old to take a stuffed animal to the hospital. When my son was only five months old, I was hospitalized for three weeks. My partner brought me a stuffed monkey that looked just like my son when he was born. It really helped me to go to sleep to have Molly the Monkey to cuddle up to. I doubt if your friends will mention it, but if they tease you, just tell them that your mother (grandmother, aunt …) gave it to you and insists that you always have it with you in the hospital.

I hate having my blood taken. This isn't good, because I have to have it done about once a month. Once I even fainted. Is there anything I can do to make it easier?

Many people have difficulty with having their blood taken. Some faint, some scream, some cry, some grit their teeth. None of these things help.

It also doesn't help when the person taking the blood tells you that it doesn't hurt that much and implies that you are acting like a baby.

Often, having blood taken *doesn't* hurt that much (unless you get the person who acts like the needle is a bulldozer and starts digging around in your arm). It is probably the idea of having something stuck into your body that is bothering you. Your skin is there to protect you, and having someone invade your body (even with something as small as a needle) can be very disturbing.

One of the best ways to deal with having blood drawn is distraction. Talk to the person who is taking the blood, or look at a picture of somewhere you would like to be and imagine you are there. *Do not look when the needle goes in!* This is essential. Ask the person who is taking the blood to tell you to take a deep breath just before she puts the needle in. (This always helps me. I'm not sure if it's because it makes me relax or if my attention is on my breathing instead of my arm.)

Don't wear anything you have to take your arm out of— make sure you can roll up the sleeve. You will feel less vulnerable if your clothes aren't half off. If the person puts the tourniquet on your bare arm, ask her to move it so it is on top of your sleeve. This way your skin won't get pinched. Make sure she lets the alcohol dry before taking your blood, or it will really sting.

If someone has tried several times and hasn't hit a vein, ask for someone else to try. Don't insult her, but be firm. *Do not bite the technician* (yes, it really has happened).

My patients who have been sexually abused have a very hard time with having blood taken. If this has been part of your experience and you don't have a therapist, get one now. She can help you work through some of your feelings, and this might help when you are having blood taken.

What drives me crazy when I'm in the hospital is that the doctors never tell me anything. I catch as much as I can on rounds, but often they talk about me and my care when I can't hear them. An aide will come to take me for a test and will seem surprised that I don't know about it. At this point, the doctors are long gone, so I can't even find out why I'm having the test.

I don't know why some doctors do this. They may think you won't understand or will ask difficult questions that they won't have the time to answer. This even happens to adults (especially old people), but it is particularly common in children's hospitals and wards. Doctors tend to be this way with young children, so if you are short for your age or for some other reason can't immediately be identified as a teen, you are more likely to be a victim of this treatment.

What you have to do is grab their attention somehow. You have to do it over and over, of course, because just when you get one set of doctors well trained, there's a whole new bunch.

Decisions about tests and procedures are usually made on morning rounds. Sometimes the doctors will ask if you have any questions, but even if they don't, there may be a pause in the yakking that is long enough to jump in and ask "Are you going to do any tests or procedures today?" If they say no, remind them to inform you if they change their minds. If they forget to do this, you may want to let them know you will not agree to any procedures unless you've been told in advance.

If you don't want to say anything this direct, consider having a large button made and always take it to the hospital with you. Use your imagination with the wording, but it could simply say "Talk to me," "I know how to communicate, let's talk," "Informed consent means I need to be informed," "What have you got planned for me?" or "Case manager in training—teach me." The advantage of this approach is that you don't have to be very assertive to use it.

Talk to a nurse about your concerns. Ask that he remind the doctors to inform you about what they want to do.

You can also ask one of your parents to talk with your doctor (often called the attending physician or staff physician) and explain how you are feeling. That doctor can in turn talk with the residents and make your wishes known.

There are a very small number of places where adults can access part of their hospital chart online. I'm not aware of any children's hospitals that are set up to do this, which is too bad.

I'm a 14-year-old guy with ulcerative colitis. My doctor is very friendly when I come to appointments and seems interested in me, not just in my disease. So I was hurt and surprised when he ignored my "friend" request on Facebook. Was I just imagining that we are friends?

In the world of social networking, it can be hard to remember that everyone who is friendly to you isn't actually your friend (and of course, some of your "friends" aren't even friendly to you!).

I'm sure your doctor likes you and is interested in you as a person. But that doesn't make him your personal friend. He might not want to friend you because he feels that it would be stepping over a boundary that does, and should, exist between you two. Doctors, ethically, aren't supposed to treat their friends and are expected to have a professional relationship with their patients. If he friends you, then you might feel hurt when he prescribes a treatment that you don't want or honestly confronts you about a concern. You might agree to a research study or treatment that you don't want because you don't want to hurt a friend.

Your doctor may want to keep his personal life and his professional life separate. Having patients as social networking friends can interfere with this. You might also not want your doctor to know some of the details about you that are in your profile or obvious from the pictures you have posted.

Communicating electronically with your health care provider can be very useful, but it is better to be done through e-mail or through a disease-related group. Ask if there is a way you can communicate electronically—some hospitals have rules against this, others want all communication to go to the patient's chart, which might not be something that you want to have happen.

My doctor is usually pretty nice, but she seems to think that everything I say and think is because I speak Spanish. She starts sentences with things like "I know your people think that ..." and "Hispanic people have been shown to ..." I don't know what makes her think she knows so much about my people. I am from a small village in Guatemala. I'm sure she's never been there. Can't she just treat me like her other patients?

Your doctor is trying to be sensitive to the differences in the ways that you may see the world (and your condition) and the ways she does. For a long time, doctors (especially white ones) have assumed that everyone comes to his or her illness with the same set of experiences, and that diversity of race, language, culture and family background do not have an impact on how people deal with their illness.

However, instead of asking you about and listening to what you have to say about your life, she is assuming you have an experience that is shared with everyone in the world who speaks Spanish. There probably are beliefs that were shared by most people in your village. They may have been shared with other Guatemalans, and even with people from other countries. But not all of them are shared.

Your doctor has shown she is willing to see that you are not exactly the same as every Anglo teen she sees. Now she needs you to help her see that you are not the same as every

Spanish-speaking person who comes to her or that she reads about.

It may be difficult for you to talk with her about this. If she says something that doesn't fit with your ideas, you might say something like "Actually, my parents think that … but I'm not sure where I stand on it." You could tell her that you don't like to be lumped with millions of other people just because you speak the same language. You can ask her if she feels she shares a common belief system with everyone who has English as a first language.

When it comes time for you to leave her care and find your own doctor, this may be an important thing to consider. You may want to devise some questions that will help you discover what their attitudes are. (For more on finding a doctor, see Chapter 8.)

I feel like the doctors and nurses here treat me like shit because I'm not some kind of perfect patient. I stayed up late, smoked dope and listened to real music before I got sick, and now they seem to think I should become a little angel or something. My goal in life is not to get onto someone's fundraising poster. It's to have a good time. Why can't they just accept this?

Health care professionals tend to like people who are easy to be around—who do what they say, don't challenge them and behave the way they want their own kids to. They may get angry with someone like you.

I think that if there are times when you feel that people are giving you bad care, are ignoring you or are treating you differently from other patients, you should talk with them about it. At the same time, you need to remember that you are dealing with human beings and that it is important to treat them as you would like to be treated (I think there's some kind of a rule about this).

Some groups, in trying to raise money, have ended up portraying kids with illnesses as "little angels." More and more, then, people come to expect this of people with disability or illness. The fact is, we all have our own personalities, and keeping them intact is one of the things we try to do in times of trouble. In addition, being in pain, feeling nauseated or just being in the hospital are all enough to make anyone crabby and not in "sweetness and light" mode.

This is a vague answer because I don't have any great ideas for changing people's attitudes. The best thing is to let them get to know you as a person and to try to get to know them. Hopefully enough people will develop more reasonable expectations as they have a chance to see you for who you are.

My doctor seems to think I'm stupid. He talks to me slowly and sometimes a bit loud. He keeps saying, "Look at me when I'm talking," but I don't feel I should be that disrespectful.

Your doctor is making an assumption about your intelligence based on body language. He has been brought up believing that people who don't look you in the eye, or who don't speak up or maybe who let their parents answer for them are not very bright. You've been brought up to believe that it is rude and disrespectful to look at adults and speak your mind to them.

Obviously, you don't want to go to a doctor and be treated as if you were stupid (and even if you were stupid, you probably wouldn't want to be addressed this way).

Can you talk with one of your parents about this? Maybe one of them could explain to him that it is important to you not to be disrespectful and that even if he doesn't view it this way, you do not want to have to change your behavior to please him. They can explain to him that you do understand what he says.

If you can't approach him this way, you may want to look for a doctor who will treat you with more respect.

> **I have a hard time remembering to take my medication. I take three different things. One pill I take just in the morning, one I take morning and night, and the other three times a day. I have a very busy life, and most of the time I don't feel too bad, so it's easy to forget. It's hard to be honest with my doctor about this because when I am, she gives me a lecture about it and I end up feeling really stupid.**

There are many reasons for people to forget their medicine. If you are feeling well, you don't have your symptoms to constantly remind you. As you point out, you can be so busy that you don't stop long enough to remember. In addition, it is easiest to remember medication if it is part of a daily routine. With a busy adolescent life, there may be few routines to link with taking your pills. Taking your pills is a three-times-a-day reminder that there is something wrong with you. Subconsciously, you may be avoiding this reminder. Whatever the reason, it isn't that you are stupid.

Here are some suggestions, both mine and those of the experts—teens who take medication.

It might be better to take your pills an hour or two earlier or later than you are supposed to if taking them at the "right" time means you will miss them frequently. Ask your doctor how important the timing of your pills is.

Sometimes a very small change in medication times can help. If you are supposed to take a pill at eight o'clock every evening but you have something you are usually doing at that time (watching a TV show, playing a video game with friends), decide that you will take your pill before that activity starts.

Try to link taking your pills to some other routine. If you always feed the dog in the morning, keep your morning pills near the dog food. Take your evening pills when you brush your teeth before going to bed.

Get a weekly pill container and dole out all your pills at the beginning of the week. If you don't want to buy one, make one out of a clean egg carton. Always make sure that your pills are not accessible to small children.

Set your watch, phone, iPod, tablet or computer to alert you to medication times.

If you don't want to carry a pill container (many are too big to go into the pockets of tight jeans), there are rings, fake watches and earrings made for younger kids that can hold pills. They have to be secure so that they don't open up unexpectedly, and you may want to carry a copy of your prescription so you can prove to suspicious adults that you don't have illicit drugs stashed in your jewelry.

Be aware that any break in routine may result in you forgetting your pills. If you go on an overnight, put your pills with your toothbrush. If you are worried that someone will see them, wrap them in your pajamas, not in the socks you'll be wearing the next day (by the time you put on your socks, you will have missed your bedtime pills).

When you go on a trip, carry two sets of pills, and pack them in different things (say, one in your purse, one in your suitcase). I was staying at a friend's cottage once and my weekly pill container fell in the toilet. I didn't have any extras with me and was lucky that I could write my own prescription and that the local drugstore had what I needed. I'll never go away without extra pills again!

There is a website called MyMedSchedule (www.mymedschedule.com) that lets you easily create a medication chart with all your medication times (you can even have it printed with pictures of the tablets or capsules). The site will remind you to take your meds with an e-mail or, if you are in the United States, a text message. In the United States there are mobile MyMedSchedule apps for both Android and Apple products.

All of your meds should be listed on your wallet-sized MyHealth Passport (www.sickkids.ca/myhealthpassport), discussed in an earlier question in this chapter.

My parents say I'm acting childish (or hysterical, that's their other favorite) because I have been trying to talk with them about how I feel about the kind of treatment I got when I was a child. I have so many memories of being held down for procedures, of having painful things done to me without any anesthetic, of hordes of people whose faces were covered with surgical masks touching me without asking. All through this, my parents just stood by and let it happen. If my parents had abused me the way people at the hospital did, I would have been taken away and put in a foster home. Why are doctors and nurses allowed to treat children that way? How can I work through these feelings and move on with my life?

For a long time, many doctors and nurses didn't try to see things from a child's point of view. They did what they felt was needed medically and didn't worry about the emotional effect it had on children. Many doctors thought that babies couldn't feel pain, so some babies even had operations without anesthetics.

Parents felt powerless. They had often been raised to think that doctors are always right. It was close to impossible for them to argue or even to question the way their children were treated.

Although there are still some very inconsiderate people around, most people who now work with children are much more respectful of them. EMLA, a local anesthetic cream that works well, is now available so that health care providers can reduce the amount of pain associated with having blood taken, lumbar punctures and other procedures. Some hospitals allow parents to accompany their children into operating rooms and stay until the procedure starts. Nurses have become more vocal in defending children. Things are far from perfect, but they are much better than when you were a child.

You are right when you say that the kind of treatment you experienced would be illegal if parents did it. You clearly carry some emotional scars. It is not uncommon for people who underwent many medical procedures as children to feel angry, to have a sense of being powerless, to experience nightmares and to have low self-esteem.

I think it would be helpful if you had a professional to talk with about this, someone who would take you seriously. Call your local child protection agency (like the CAS, the Children's Aid Society) and ask for names of therapists who are good with teens who were abused when they were younger. You may want to ask your parents to come with you after you have found a therapist you like. They may be denying the effect your treatment had on you because they feel guilty that they didn't stick up for you.

The last time I was in the hospital, I shared a room with another teen. He had a problem that meant he couldn't talk very well. He couldn't get across what he wanted to say. Like me, he had to go for lots of tests. A few times, when he came back, he was obviously upset but couldn't tell me why. I noticed that when a certain staff member took him for his tests, he always came back upset. This happened right before I went home, and he kept on pointing to his penis. I didn't do anything. Should I do anything now? Is this all my imagination?

I'm sure you didn't imagine all this. You don't know what happened to your roommate, but you know something got him upset, and that it was always after he was with a certain person.

People do get abused (physically, verbally and sexually) in hospitals and institutions. The vast majority of people who work in hospitals are not abusers. Abusers pick on people who they think won't or can't tell about what is happening to them. They pick victims who already feel bad about themselves and try to leave them with the feeling that what happened is the victim's fault.

It is not too late to do something about this. You or one of your parents should call the hospital and find out if it has a patient representative or patient advocate. If it does, call and talk to this person. Tell her all you know about the situation. If there is no one like this at the hospital, you or your parent can talk to a nursing supervisor. It is important for this matter to be investigated.

What can you do to protect yourself from people like this? The most important thing is to be sure within yourself that no one has the right to treat you that way, and if anyone—a porter, a nurse, a doctor, a neighbor, a relative—touches you in a way that you don't like or that hurts or that you feel is wrong, tell the person to stop, and tell someone about it. Even if the person threatens you, tell someone. If you can't talk, then scream, point at the person and do everything you can not to go anywhere alone with that person.

Most people who are abused are hurt by people they know and would have reason to trust—parents, other relatives or family friends. One of the reasons for this is that, in general, young people aren't alone with people who aren't known to them. Children and teens who have health conditions or disabilities are more likely to be in vulnerable situations in hospitals, in educational settings and while being transported. Keeping an eye out will help you protect yourself and those around you who may not be able to speak for themselves.

Every time I go to the doctor, he goes on and on about what is wrong with me. He says that I should know everything about my illness so that I can make good decisions and be more in control of things. I don't want these constant reminders of what is wrong with me. When he doesn't bring it up, I can just go along, feeling normal.

There is a very fine balance here, one that for you must be like walking a tightrope.

When you feel constantly reminded about your condition, it makes you feel like a sick person, as if your illness is the main part of who you are. I'm sure it makes you feel that your illness is more important to your doctor than you are. Some amount of pretending to yourself and others that there is nothing wrong with you can be helpful in achieving a normal lifestyle.

On the other hand, if you don't have any sense of having a chronic condition, you will be less likely to take your medication, go for appointments or do other things to keep yourself healthy.

In addition, if you do not have adequate information about your condition, the best you can do is pretend it doesn't exist. If you are more knowledgeable, you may get to a point where you actually feel in control of it—a very powerful feeling.

One possibility is to tell your doctor how you are feeling. Maybe you could stand to be educated on half your visits, or a third of them. Let him know what kind of information would be helpful to you (maybe about sex). Ask that it be given in a positive manner. You may want all the information you get for a while to be aimed specifically at helping you become more independent.

I'm sure that your doctor will be willing to tone down a bit. He knows that he can't make you learn anything you don't want to. In a way, you are lucky. Many teens complain that their doctors won't tell them anything, and that they know very little about their conditions.

When I go to the clinic, I see a bunch of different medical people. Not only am I involved with different kinds of doctors, I hardly ever see the real specialists. It is usually just an intern or a resident whom I've never met before, and who wants to hear my entire life history. I've been thinking of writing it down and giving it to them. I feel like there is no one in charge, and I would like there to be. Is this asking too much?

I think you deserve to have someone coordinating your care. This doesn't mean never seeing a resident, but it would involve having someone responsible for your care and making sure that things happen in an organized fashion. You would have someone you could approach with questions and concerns.

This job has frequently been given the name "case manager." Nurses, clinical nurse specialists and nurse-practitioners often take on this role, but if most of your contact is with physicians, then it would make sense for it to be a doctor.

Think about the specialists you have seen. Is there one with whom you feel you communicate well, someone who respects you and is willing to listen to what you have to say? If so, it would make sense to ask this person to be your case manager and to coordinate your care at the clinic and if you have to be admitted to the hospital. Assure her that you understand you will still be seeing residents but that you would like a few minutes with her when you have appointments.

If there is no one with whom you have a bond, you can either ask the specialist who you see most often to be your case manager, or ask if they have a fellow or other trainee who will be around for a year or two who could do the job. Fellows are fully trained specialists (in your case, they are usually pediatricians) who are being trained as subspecialists. Although having a fellow as a case manager means you will have to find a new one in a couple of years, he might be quite eager to become this involved and to put some time into the relationship. And you never know, the person may end up staying on as a staff doctor at the end of his training. There may be a team at your hospital that takes care of teenagers (this specialty is called adolescent medicine). One of these people may be willing to be a case manager and could also have information about things like birth control, sex, drugs and other teenage concerns.

Make a MyHealth Passport and practice a three-sentence summary (both discussed earlier in the chapter). You need to say when you were diagnosed, what your diagnosis is, whether you have had any surgical procedures and what drugs you are currently taking. You can print an extra MyHealth Passport to go into your chart, but bring your copy with you to appointments so if the chart copy gets lost, you have a backup.

My doctor never asked me how I felt about having really big breasts. It couldn't be that he didn't notice, because they are huge. I talked to him about it yesterday. I told him about how self-conscious I feel, how I walk hunched over to try to hide them. I told him how I have to wear a bra all the time, and how the straps are wearing ruts into my shoulders. He said that lots of girls would be happy to have breasts like mine. He told me it would be foolish for me to have reduction surgery for something like this when I have had to undergo operations for my illness and may need more. I felt really stupid.

You weren't stupid. You were brave to bring this up, and it is too bad that he wasn't able to respond appropriately.

Despite the fact that a small number of women have operations to give them enormous breasts, most women feel uncomfortable with breasts that are much larger than average. For one thing, there is the physical discomfort of back pain and poor posture. But more important is the emotional discomfort. Men tend to stare at women and girls who have large breasts. People may even make rude comments.

It sounds as though you have had many operations that you didn't have much choice about. It is important for you to be able to make a choice about this. Having had other operations means that you have a more realistic picture of what surgery really involves than someone else your age might. You know about how you feel when you wake up from an operation, that things do not always go as planned, that your idea of a perfect result and that of the surgeon's might be different.

Talk with one of your parents and get him or her on your side. Make sure your parent understands that what you want is information about your options. If neither of them supports you in this, you will have to pursue it on your own, but it would be helpful to have their support. Take a parent with you and see one of your other doctors. If it wasn't your family doctor who was so insensitive, he or she is probably your best bet. You should be able to get a referral to a plastic surgeon who has experience with teens.

When you see the plastic surgeon, ask your parent to take notes, and get as much information as you can about what you can expect as a final outcome, how long it will take to recover, and what the possible complications are, including any long-term ones. You want to end up with nipples that have normal sensation and with the ability to breast-feed. Then go home and think about it. Don't be swayed by a surgeon who is too optimistic and glosses over the possibility of problems.

If you decide to have surgery, chances are you will have a good outcome and be happy with the result. Your original doctor will find out about this at some point, and if you are up to it, you may want to let him know that his answer to you when you first brought up the topic wasn't helpful. You can let him know that even if "most girls" would be happy with large breasts (which I doubt), you weren't and you weren't asking him about most girls.

I have sickle cell anemia, and when I have a crisis, I am in excruciating pain. Usually, I go to the hospital emergency room and get painkillers right away. Last week when I was visiting relatives who live in a small town, I started having bad stomach pains. I went to the local hospital. When I told the doctor what my usual dose is (I had it written down for just this kind of situation) he said that it was way too high, and that I would become addicted if I kept taking that much. The amount he gave me didn't really help, and my parents had to drive me back to the city. What can I do to prevent this from happening again, other than never going away?

I can see how you might be scared to leave the city after this, but it is important not to be imprisoned by your condition.

Many doctors have been taught in medical school to be highly cautious with narcotic painkillers, and for good reason. People with minor or short-term problems have been given too much or kept on them too long and have ended up addicted. But this healthy fear of narcotics has made some doctors so paranoid that they don't want to prescribe strong painkillers when they should. They may be especially reluctant to use them when the patient is young or is unknown to them. In addition, if you are black, you may have been faced with racial prejudice. The doctor may have been feeling that black people are more likely to use or abuse drugs and therefore denied what you need.

In addition to carrying a MyHealth Passport (www.sick-kids.ca/myhealthpassport), get a wallet-sized piece of heavy paper. Ask your doctor to write on it your dosage and that you are not addicted. Have her sign and date this, and include her phone number. Then get it laminated in a laminating machine—you can often find one in bus or train station, or try a mall. Carry this card with you in your wallet at all times. It may help convince someone if you are ever in this situation again. If the doctor still refuses to give you the correct amount of painkillers, ask him or her to call your doctor. If the doctor doesn't want to do this, get to a pay phone and call your doctor. Ask her to call the person who is denying you proper treatment.

Contact the MedicAlert Foundation and ask if you can update your information whenever your dose is increased. Then, if you are faced with someone who doesn't believe you and your doctor can't be reached, the person can get in touch with MedicAlert (the phone number is on your bracelet).

When my doctor takes blood from me, she always puts on gloves. All this time she's been telling me that what I have isn't catching. Has she been telling the truth? She can't be doing it just to keep her hands clean. I mean, she could wash them, couldn't she?

Many hospitals have switched over to something called "universal precautions." Among other things, this means that people wear gloves when they might come into contact with blood. The reason for this is that you can't tell by looking at someone if he or she has a condition like hepatitis or HIV that could be passed on if blood got into a cut or scrape. So we now act as though everyone has something infectious.

Only a small number of people do have a condition that is passed along this way, so lots of gloves are used when they aren't really needed. But since there is no good way to know which patients to wear gloves with and which not to, this is a good compromise. Also, it would single out people with something infectious if doctors used gloves only for them. Everyone would know who they were, and they might end up being treated differently in other ways.

As well, when your doctor wears gloves, she is protecting you from germs on her hands.

If your condition was catching, your doctor would tell you, so that you could protect those around you. I think you can trust her on this one. You may want to ask her to explain to her patients why she uses gloves so that other people don't have to worry the way you did.

I have a lot of trouble falling asleep at night. Then the next day I feel horrible. My doctor won't give me a sleeping pill; he says I could get addicted. Is there anything else I can do?

What you can do has a lot to do with what is causing your problem. Many teens have difficulty falling asleep. The reason may be related to your condition, or it could be something else.

One thing to look at is what you consume, medication and otherwise. For instance, caffeine intake can also lead to sleep difficulties. How much caffeine are you taking in? Remember that there is caffeine in soft drinks, chocolate bars, wake-up pills and some headache medications, as well as in coffee and tea. In general, it is a good idea to stay away from anything with caffeine in it after supper time: there is no set cut-off time for caffeine intake, but very few people can consume it at or after supper and still fall asleep easily. Consider avoiding foods containing caffeine (including brown soft drinks, energy drinks, coffee, black or green tea and chocolate) for a few days to see if it makes a difference.

Some medications can cause sleep problems. Ritalin and other drugs that are used for attention deficit disorder often make it difficult to sleep, and you may want to talk with your doctor about changing the medication or the times you take it. Drugs used to treat depression can also result in sleep problems. You should check with your doctor to see if any of your medications might be leading to your problem. Street drugs like speed and cocaine can interfere with sleep. Although alcohol may make you drowsy, some people find that they wake up in the middle of the night when they have been drinking.

Some conditions are associated with problems sleeping. Pain can keep you up at night. Taking your medications regularly might help control the pain. Your doctor might be able to change your pain medication or timing to help you sleep. Masturbating at bedtime can sometimes relieve pain and help sleep. Some people who have had a brain injury have a hard time falling asleep, as do people with fibromyalgia. A drug called amitriptyline is used in small doses to help people with both of these conditions sleep. Teens who are visually impaired also report sleep problems. This is because the brain is triggered by cycles of light and darkness to produce chemicals that regulate sleep. Some blind teens have been helped by a hormone called melatonin. This is available in pill form at health food stores. Because it is not well regulated, different brands have varying effectiveness. Some pills, when tested, didn't even have any melatonin in them! You might be able to find a review in a publication like *Consumer Reports* that tells you which brands are the best. People who are on some immunosuppressant medications shouldn't take melatonin—talk to a health care practitioner about melatonin and your meds.

Both depression and anxiety can cause sleep problems. Although some people with depression sleep much more than usual, or wake up very early in the morning, many depressed teens say they have difficulty falling asleep at night. Lying in bed and worrying is not something that helps people sleep. Try to make a plan for something good to think about as you fall asleep, like what you would do with a million dollars, or remembering a great vacation.

If you aren't already talking with someone about how you are feeling, you should strongly consider doing this. Your doctor or nurse may be able to counsel you or, if not, should be able to recommend a counselor or therapist. Although I said above that depression medication can cause sleep problems, many teens who are on them sleep much better. If you've experienced trauma (like being sexually abused or seeing something awful happen), you need to tell someone about it and get some counseling.

People who specialize in sleep problems talk a lot about what they call "sleep hygiene." They feel that the events that happen in your life, particularly in the evening, can have a real impact on sleep. They suggest that you get some exercise every day, but not do any vigorous exercise in the hour or two before sleep. They say you shouldn't eat after supper, other than a snack about half an hour before bedtime that is low in fat and has milk as part of it. A bath that is warm but not too hot before bedtime can also help. They recommend not having a television in your bedroom, avoiding computer use in your bed and shutting off your phone at night (even having it set to vibrate can wake you when you get a text message).

You can try all or some of these things. I would particularly recommend regular exercise. It might not help right away, but after a couple of weeks, it is likely you will see a big improvement in your sleep.

3 Friends and Dating

THIS CHAPTER ANSWERS a number of questions about getting and keeping friends, and about dating. Time spent "out of circulation" because of being in the hospital or at home sick can make it harder to make friends and maintain friendships, but it can be done. If you are lucky, some of the friends you make now will be with you for the rest of your life.

> **When a guy who doesn't know about my illness asks me out, do I have to tell him before we go out, on the first date, when things get serious or when? I don't wear a MedicAlert bracelet, and other than being too thin, my illness isn't noticeable. I don't want to scare anyone off, but I hate to be dishonest.**

You have no obligation to tell anyone you are dating or want to date about your disease at a particular time. Obviously, if you end up in a relationship with this person, you don't want a secret hanging over your head. On the other hand, it may be a good idea to let someone get to know you as a person so that when he finds out about your illness it's only one of many things he knows about you. If your illness or medication is going to affect what you can do, then it becomes more important that you tell him. You don't have to be specific right away. Saying something like "I can't drink because of the medication I'm on" is fine. If you are very secretive, it will affect how he sees you as a person.

He may guess that you are hiding something and may imagine that it is something terrible.

The exception to the "no obligation to tell" rule is that if you are HIV positive, you should, and may be legally required to tell the other person before you have sex with them. Even if you always use a condom, it could break and they would be at risk.

I would encourage you to wear a Medic Alert bracelet. They can be crucial in an emergency. Lots of kids wear them because of allergies or because they wear contact lenses. If someone asks you why you wear it, you can always say it's because you are allergic to people who ask personal questions. Another possibility is to wear a MedicAlert necklace. You can keep the pendant tucked inside your shirt, and all that will be visible will be the chain.

Whether or not you wear a MedicAlert bracelet, necklace or watch, you should consider making a MyHealth Passport, a wallet-sized card with your important health information (see the Resources section for more information on this). It is unlikely that a guy you have just started seeing will be going through your wallet (if he does, he isn't a keeper), so the information will be private but available in an emergency.

I want to use Facebook to connect with other people with my condition. It is pretty rare and there isn't a Facebook group for it. But I'm not sure that I want my other friends to see my connection to my disease. I've thought a lot about this and I am not ready to let them know about it. How can I manage this?

Social networking is a great way to find other people who have a rare disease. Remember that there is no way to verify that everyone in the group has the condition, so just like with your other social networking, don't be entirely trusting.

As secrecy is important to you, I would suggest using a different site—Facebook isn't the only one out there. You can even create your own social network. Currently, the most commonly used site for doing this is Ning.

Getting the word out, particularly on a lesser-known or new network, is going to be your challenge. I would suggest that you set it up and then let your nurse or nurse-practitioner know that you have done this and how people can join the group. You might even make up a flyer and ask them to e-mail it to their colleagues or take it to a conference. Those people can pass it on to their patients. They won't be giving you any information about these people, so their privacy will be protected.

There might also be a lower-tech solution to go along with this. There will be a national or international conference that your healthcare team goes to that deals with your disease (or a group of diseases that it fits into). Ask if they have a component for young people at the conferences. If not, you can encourage them to start this. Many conferences do include "consumers," including that of the World Federation of Hemophilia and the annual North American Cystic Fibrosis Conference (NACFC). While these conferences aren't on rare conditions, they set an example of what can be done, so the organization dealing with your condition won't have to invent a model from scratch.

My best friend and I spend almost all of our spare time together. We walk home from school together (we're in Grade 7), join the same clubs, work together on projects and talk on the phone for hours. My mother says I'm cutting myself off from other

people. She says I am scared that other people won't like me because of my illness, so I don't even try. It doesn't feel this way to me. Should I go along with her and try to make other friends?

It often bothers parents when their young teens seem to get totally absorbed in a friendship. It can be hard for them to understand how important it is to have a best friend.

Having a close friend is the best practice you can get for adult relationships. You are learning to be intimate with someone you aren't related to. You can talk about things that worry you that would be embarrassing to reveal to your parents. You try out different ways of behaving and communicating (not to mention different hairstyles and clothes). Rather than limiting you, your friendship should help you feel more comfortable being with people your own age.

When is a friendship going too far? When you or your friend feel jealous if the other one talks with someone else or spends time with another person. When one person controls the other's behavior or gets all the attention in the friendship. When someone keeps the friendship going by making the other person feel bad. From your description, none of these things are part of your friendship.

Your mother may be feeling a bit jealous as you confide more in your friend and less in her. She may be feeling that she never gets to see you or talk to you.

Try spending a bit of time every day (if your family eats together, supper is a good time for this) showing an interest in your mother and what she is doing.

See if you and your friend can spend some time with a larger group of kids, maybe some other best friends whose parents are also putting pressure on them. Talk about these other kids around your mother so that she knows you are socializing with them. In addition to making her feel better, you will benefit from having a wider circle of friends without losing your important "best friendship."

> **I am 17 and have been realizing over the past few years that I am much more attracted to other girls than to boys. I'm starting to feel OK about this, I think, and I know that I'm not the only person to feel this way. A (male) friend of mine at school recently told me he is gay. He's worried because he says how you look is really important in the gay community, and he doesn't think he's attractive enough. Is there any place for someone like me, with a chronic illness, in what seems like such an exclusive community? Am I doomed to be alone all my life?**

No, of course not.

To start with, the large numbers of gays and lesbians make it impossible for there to be one "right" way to be gay. Second, the men's and women's communities are different entities. Many gay men have placed a fairly high value on physical appearance in the past. Many gay males, however, do not fit the stereotype of an attractive gay man, but they still had relationships. The gay community has matured over the last 20 years as it has had to deal with the AIDS crisis, and my perception is that now there is more attention paid to who people are rather than how they look.

The lesbian community is made up of many different groups of women. The most visible of these are women who are politically active. Because many come from a feminist perspective, they have emphasized inclusion and trying to encompass all lesbians with a similar philosophy.

Being a lesbian with a chronic condition or disability is probably not any easier than being a heterosexual in the same situation. You will meet lesbians who are interested only in women who look, act or dress a certain way. You will meet other lesbians who are interested in who you are and in your thoughts and feelings. You may encounter some discrimination from certain lesbians, but you're also likely to find yourself welcomed and included by many others.

Some people might suggest that you check out the It Gets Better Project, which has thousands of recordings of people talking about how difficult it was to be young and gay and then things got better. This is an important project, aiming to reach out to young people who might become suicidal as a result of being bullied or treated badly because people know or think they are gay. However, its purpose isn't to reflect the experiences of young people who haven't had a hard time, so it can give the impression that teen life will be awful for you. When I searched for "disability" on the site, there wasn't anything helpful, but when I went to a different search engine, I did find one amazing video by a Costa Rican teen who talks about being bullied because of his disability and how coming out as gay helped others see him as a person, not just a disability.

If you live in a big city, there is probably a group for disabled lesbians that would include people with chronic illnesses. Get in touch with it for more information. A gay youth group would be another good place to start. If you live in a smaller town, things are tougher. It is often hard to find out where other lesbians your age hang out. Check the Yellow Pages. There might be a listing for a gay hotline under "homosexuality," "gay" or "lesbian."

I was really interested in a guy in my math class a couple of months ago, but I felt pretty discouraged about it. I use a wheelchair, and somehow, this seems to get the boys thinking of me as a pal

rather than a girlfriend. My best friend encouraged me to talk to him and to try to get him interested. She was very supportive. It worked, and I've been going out with Mike most weekends and we walk home from school together a few days a week. Now my friend is complaining that she doesn't see me enough, and that when we are together all I do is talk about him. Why has she become so unsupportive?

I think you need to look at this from her point of view. She was being a good, supportive friend when she encouraged you to get to know Mike better. She wasn't asking you to desert her, and that's what she feels you've done.

You are going through what many young women experience with their first boyfriend. It is somewhat magnified, as you seemed to feel before that you would never attract someone because of your disability. This relationship is taking up a fair bit of your time. Try to remember that your friend might be feeling abandoned.

You do not need to stop seeing Mike to save your friendship. When you are with your friend, focus on being with her. Limit the amount of time you spend talking about Mike. Don't pretend he doesn't exist, but don't make him the center of all discussions. Set aside some time most weekends to get together with her to shop, study, listen to music, or whatever you used to do.

Friendships are precious and tend to have a longer life span than romantic relationships, but they do need some care. Don't lose a good friend through neglect.

I am 16 and have a tracheostomy (a hole in my neck to breathe through), and a lot of the time I am hooked up to a ventilator. I can go to school, to

concerts, whatever, but I always have to have an "attendant" with me. There is a nurse who goes to school with me, but the rest of the time, that person is one of my parents. It gets a bit awkward. I know my parents can't afford an attendant—if they could, I'm sure they would love to go out on a date sometimes and leave me at home with someone who could take care of the trach.

Having a parent or nurse with you all the time can really cramp your style, even when you get along well, which it sounds like you do.

Do you have one or two close friends who would be willing to be trained in trach care? It can be learned, and I know of teens who have done this. The main thing is that they have to get past feeling scared about this.

If you can identify some people, e-mail your nurse-practitioner or whoever is your contact person for your trach/ ventilator care and tell them you have found someone to do your trach care. If they seem reluctant to let a teen do trach care, show them this page of this book so that they can see that it is being done in other places.

My suggestion would be to not have someone in whom you are romantically interested be one of these helpers. Once you are in a serious relationship, the person you are with will need to know how to do this, but providing physical care for you might not be the best way to get them thinking romantically about you.

My best friend is reading a book about self-esteem. She says she thinks mine is terrible, probably because of being sick so much. What is self-esteem, anyway? How can I tell if she is right?

Self-esteem is how you feel about who you are and what you can do. If it is low, you have a low value of your worth as a human being; if it is high, you feel good about yourself.

There is no formula for developing high self-esteem. We know that people who feel accepted for who they are and who have seen that others value them tend to have high self-esteem. You can have high self-esteem with any kind of chronic condition. If you feel your condition is your fault, or if it has stopped you from succeeding in some important way, this can contribute to low self-esteem.

Why is self-esteem important? It has a huge impact on how you perform in a variety of activities. If you think you aren't worth much, you won't do as well as if you know you can succeed. High self-esteem helps when you are making friends. If people pick up on the fact that you feel good about yourself, they will see you as someone worth knowing. High self-esteem will aid you in staying healthy. You are more likely to take care of yourself if you feel you have some value. Low self-esteem may make you vulnerable to exploitation or abuse in a relationship. You may feel that you deserve to be treated badly.

Here are some ways you can judge what your self-esteem is like. Listen to what you say about yourself. Do you frequently complain that you are too fat or too thin? Do you start sentences with statements like "I'm probably wrong, but …"? Sit down with a piece of paper and write down what you like about yourself and what you think you are good at. If you can't think of anything, then you have low self-esteem.

If you find that your feelings about yourself are negative, you aren't stuck with this forever. Ask your friend what she thinks are your good points. Make a list of these things and add things you think of yourself. Look at the list every morning. If you do well in something, let yourself feel good about it. If you catch yourself starting to say something to put yourself down, stop. Stay quiet for a minute instead. If there are things you enjoy doing and are good at, do them more often. If there aren't, start looking for some new activities that you can succeed at.

I'm 16 and I'm only 5 feet 3 inches tall. I'll probably get to be a bit taller, but I feel like a runt. The guys at school seem so sure of themselves, they know how to act, they're tough and self-confident. When I try to act that way, I feel I'm faking it. They're the real men (well, almost men). I don't come close.

I want to let you in on men's biggest secret: No teenaged boy or young man thinks he's a real man deep down inside—at least I've never met any who do. My brother tells a story of learning how to smoke "like a guy," how to stand, how to hold the cigarette… Men who feel comfortable with their identities don't have to go around acting like they're tough, always strong and in control. They don't need to put down girls or other guys. They can shed a tear, be vulnerable, you know, just be human beings—confident some times and hopeless the next.

When you are with your friends, notice which ones seem to have to prove something and which ones do not.

By definition, you're a man. And the truth is, you don't need to prove that to anyone.

I don't see how I will make any friends while I am fat. My mother says I am a beautiful person and that someday people will see that and not judge me just on how I look, but I don't think I can wait. I tried to stop eating but it is so hard with the steroids that I take for my lupus. What can I do?

It is true that many teens (and even adults) judge people by how they look and that body weight is one of the things that influences these judgments. Many teens who are average weight try to lose weight because they feel fat. Many of those who do lose weight do not find that they have more friends or are more popular. Even if you are being bullied about your weight, losing weight is not a guarantee that the bullying will stop. Bullies are looking for vulnerable people and will often find a new soft spot to harass you about.

It is awful to be excluded or to feel that you have no friends, and I'm sure you'd like to find the reason this is happening to you and fix it. It may be that some of what you are going through is because of your weight. But starving yourself is not the answer.

New research shows that young people who take steroids for lupus are unlikely to end up obese by the time they are off the steroids—about 10% become obese. One of the things that makes steroid weight gain so difficult to cope with is that it shows in your face so much. This is an effect that goes away as your dose is lowered.

You should talk with the dietician at your clinic and find out if you are overweight and by how much. She can help you adjust what you are eating so that you can gradually lose weight. If you have been gaining steadily, even holding your weight steady would be an improvement. She will probably recommend that you increase your intake of vegetables and fruits, and decrease or cut out fried foods, donuts and other fast-food items. When you make changes in what you eat, you want to see results quickly. But it isn't healthy to lose the weight quickly. If you are overweight, losing a pound or two a week is more realistic and better for you. So it might take six months or longer before you reach your goal. You will need support through this process.

Increasing your exercise will help you lose weight and will also help you feel better about yourself and your capabilities. You may also be able to find someone who would like to walk, swim or do another activity with you, and perhaps develop a friendship with them.

When I got kidney disease, my friends were great. They visited me at the hospital and gave me copies of their notes so I wouldn't get too far behind in school. Things have remained OK at school, but two of my friends don't invite me over after school anymore. I finally asked one of them about this and she said her parents said she couldn't be my friend because she might catch what I have. She explained that it's not contagious, but they don't believe her. Is there anything I can do about this situation? I don't have a huge group of friends, so I can't just spend time with other people instead.

This is a difficult situation and it illustrates one of the hardest things about being a teen with a chronic condition—the ignorance of many people with whom you come into contact. Dealing with ignorant adults is not as simple as educating them. Most will not believe you because you're "only a kid."

Ask your doctor for any pamphlets that show your disease is not contagious. If none are available from your doctor, write to the Kidney Foundation to see if it has anything. (For teens in this situation who have a different condition: Most diseases have a foundation. Your doctor should be able to give you the address or some information about the one for your condition.)

If you can get such a pamphlet, give copies to these friends to give to their parents.

If you can't find a pamphlet, think about writing a letter to the parents explaining that your disease is not catching and explaining a bit about it. Ask your doctor to sign the letter, using as many official-looking letters after his name as he is entitled to use.

It sounds as though your friends still do things with you at school, but if they don't, I wonder if it really is your friends and not their parents who are fearful. Sometimes people blame their parents for things they themselves don't want to do. If they are avoiding you at school, it is important to make sure they understand that they can't catch your illness.

I really want to be involved with someone. I try being really friendly to people, but it doesn't seem to work. I have some friends of both sexes, and I try to meet lots of people so that someone will be attracted to me and fall in love with me. I don't know if it is my disability or something else that is getting in the way, but I'm getting desperate.

Your desperation may be the problem. It is a sad fact of life that when a person seems very anxious to meet someone and fall in love, it tends to scare people off. Maybe they feel that you don't really care who that someone is but that anyone will do. Most people don't want to be treated like interchangeable parts. Your eagerness may also be overwhelming. Despite the images in soap operas and romance novels, most people do not fall in love at first sight. They need time to develop a relationship.

I worry that you want this so badly that you will get involved with whoever expresses an interest in you, whether or not you actually like the person or are compatible with him or her.

A person doesn't need to have an illness or disability to be in your position. For every happy couple you see at the movies, there are 20 teenagers at home wishing they had a date or are out with friends and feeling that what they have is second best. It isn't, of course. A real relationship, as opposed to a brief fling, is built on friendship and common interests.

Don't look for romance at every turn. Spend time with the friends you have now, having fun and learning more about them. Notice what is going on in your community and the world at large. Conversation can go far beyond what the school basketball team is doing. (This doesn't mean that your conversations should sound like the evening news or lectures on the state of the world. Discuss news items that mean something to you, that touch your life.) Be honest about your disability. If you can be matter-of-fact about it and clear about any special needs you have, your friends (and prospective romantic partners) will feel comfortable being with you. Although it is OK to complain sometimes, don't be a broken record, whining about how unfair life is. This will not attract anyone.

Consider getting a weekend job—it is a great way to meet new people. If jobs are scarce in your community or your parents don't want you to work at this time, volunteer for a community organization. This could be a political campaign, an environmental group, an AIDS support project, a food bank, a non-profit day-care center or something similar. There are numerous possibilities, and in all of them you will meet new people, but more importantly, your life will be full.

Be wary of meeting people online. I'm not aware of any safe dating sites for people under 18. If you meet someone through a social networking site, you can end up feeling that you know them very well before you meet them. But this doesn't mean that you can trust them. If you want to meet someone whom you've met online, make sure you go with a friend (preferably of the opposite sex) and that you have told someone else where you are going and who you are meeting. Make the meeting happen in a public place. Even if it goes well, wait to meet the person alone until he or she has hung out with your friends and you a number of times.

Sooner or later you will fall in love with someone. But it may not be soon, so don't plan your life around it.

You would think that teasing is something for little kids, but I find that I still get tormented about how I look, especially if I'm not with friends. It scares me to be the object of this hostility (I refuse to believe that they are "just kidding"). Am I being paranoid?

I have to agree with you about that. As far as I can tell, there are two reasons why people tease. The first is that they are scared. They may have been brought up in families where it is normal to be afraid of anyone who is different. Or, when confronted by your condition, it reminds them that "bad" things happen to people, and they react against you because they are psychologically fending off this reminder.

Second, they may get their kicks by exerting power over someone else. They may come from a family where one of their parents, in order to feel stronger, picks on the kids. People like this will pick on anyone who seems vulnerable, either because they are physically different from the norm, come from a different kind of family, are open about a homosexual orientation or are from a religious, ethnic or racial minority.

Dealing with this can be difficult. The traditional advice of ignoring them or not showing them that you are upset will work much of the time, but it may leave you feeling powerless. Also, they may try more and more to get you upset, and this could extend to a physical assault. A more sophisticated version of this approach is to look the person in the eye, and say, "I refuse to be treated like this." By looking them in eye, you have forced them to make some kind of contact. They can save face by saying that they were just kidding.

A snappy comeback will often work with the person who is afraid or ignorant, but it may be seen as a challenge to the person who is looking for power. Also, if they live with a person who uses sarcasm to get power over them, they may see your snappy comeback in that light and again get violent. If you don't feel there's much hostility in the situation, the comic approach may be your best choice.

If you are in a public place, it is usually safe to just leave the situation. You need to view this as taking positive action rather than as running away. However, if there is no one around, you might be chased or even caught.

If you do feel that there is a danger of physical assault, shout repeatedly at the top of your lungs, "I'm being assaulted! Call 911!"

Last week, a guy in one of my classes asked me where I had been (I was admitted to the hospital for a few weeks). We chatted for a few minutes and then his girlfriend came over and said, "Hands off, he's mine." I explained that we were just chatting, and I thought the incident was over. She friended me on Facebook later that day, which I thought was her way of apologizing for overreacting. But the next day she was writing on my wall about how "nasty" I am and calling me names. She even posted photos of prostitutes and tagged them with my name!

Social networking has been a great way for people to connect, but it has also been a way for bullies to extend their power. Contact the Facebook administrators about the tagging, since there is nothing you on your own can do to change this.

Tell your friends this is happening and why, so that they can watch for other instances of cyber-bullying from her. (And while you are at it, unfriend the person who did the tagging.)

In general, there are things that you can do to make your social networking experience safer. To start with, accept only real friends as Facebook friends. If you do accept someone other than close friends, give them very limited access. This goes for all types of social networking, not just Facebook.

Strangers can bully you just as easily as someone you have met. Check your security settings regularly, as they may get changed with minimal notice to you. Even with very tight restrictions, people have been able to get very private information and photos. Don't post anything that you wouldn't want your parents or an employer to see.

Limit the amount of personal information, and don't post your phone number or address.

Never give your password to anyone, not even your best friend. Don't respond to any messages that claim to be from a bank, credit card company or contest and ask you to enter your password. When setting a password, make it long and a mixture of letters and numbers. Don't use your name or date of birth as a password.

I thought my social life would improve as I got older, but it seems to be getting worse. In junior high I had a few friends who lived in apartments and would invite me to their place after school or come to mine. Now I'm in Grade 12, and only one of those

**friends is at my school. I have friends at school
who I eat lunch with, but I never see them outside of school. I'm sure that my wheelchair scares
them off. What can I do to change this?**

The move to high school changes many teens' available
friendships. At the beginning of the year, most of the people
you see every day are strangers. By the end of Grade 9, many
people have found new friends with the same interests.

The kids you grew up with learned to see you as a person
and probably didn't notice your wheelchair any more than they
would notice someone's glasses or hair color. In high school,
many of the people you see on a daily basis have never had a
friend in a chair. They may feel intimidated by it and worry
that you couldn't get around easily in their homes (if you can
even get into the house). You may notice that people seem to
be more cautious about what they say to you than they are with
others.

High school can be a very lonely time, and the feelings that
you are having could lead to depression, so I think you are right
to want to change things.

First, I think you need to think about what kind of image
you project. Do you see yourself as a severely disabled person?
If you do, then you are probably projecting this to other people.
Try to start viewing yourself as healthier. When you are with
other people, make sure that you listen to what they are saying,
and show that you are doing this by looking at them, nodding
occasionally, and asking questions that show you are interested.
You may have been feeling a bit desperate and talking too
much. I'm not telling you to never talk or to never mention
your disability. I'm just saying you need to make sure you aren't
always trying to be the center of attention.

Are your transportation arrangements getting in the way of hanging out after school? If you don't drive and don't live close enough to school to get home by yourself, consider getting your ride to come later to get you. If nothing is happening, you can always study in the library.

Consider joining a club after school so that you can meet people with the same interests. It may then be an easier step to invite them to your house to see a relevant computer program that you have, say, or something else relating to your mutual interest. If you think it may be a bit scary for kids to invite you home, see if you can arrange something more casual, like going with a bunch of them to the mall after school.

If your junior high friend has friends she sees outside of school who are also school friends of yours or are people you would like to get to know better, consider asking her to invite one or two of them over after school or on a weekend when you will be there. It may break the ice with some people if they can see it isn't a big deal to have you over.

You may have been excluding other people in chairs from your group of potential friends because you are worried that others will think you only want friends with a similar disability. Don't be too quick to do this, as there may be some great people wheeling around your school that you've been ignoring.

Through some friends at my school I met a girl who goes to another school. She seemed really great and interested in me. I often feel that my wheelchair gets in the way of girls seeing me as interesting in the way I'd like them to be. Getting to know her on a social networking site helped her see past my disability, or so I thought. When we were going to meet, she asked, "How can I know

I can trust you?" I gave her my password so that she would know that she was seeing everything I posted. The next thing I knew, she shared it with some other people and they changed things on my wall in a really hurtful way. When I asked her why she had done this, she said, "I just couldn't resist— it made me feel like I had so much power. I didn't think they would do anything mean."

Hopefully you were able to change your password and get back control of your information—I've talked to young people who have had their online identity totally hijacked. You aren't alone. It has been shown that up to one-third of teens in relationships have given their password as a sign of trust. It doesn't always end badly, but it can. You've learned the hard way never to give your password to anyone. Even if you have already met the person, are dating or in a long-term relationship. Even if it is your best friend.

I wouldn't assume that what she did means that she was malicious or never really interested in you. It sounds more like she is very immature and acts without thinking. Don't take this as a sign that no one will want to be with you for yourself.

To protect yourself from identity theft, don't respond to any messages that claim to be from a bank, credit card company or contest and ask you to enter your password. When setting a password, make it long and a mixture of letters and numbers. Don't use your name or date of birth as a password. One way to keep an eye on whether anyone is pretending to be you is to sign up for a free alert service, such as Google Alerts, that will search automatically for your name showing up on the Internet. You can set how often you want this to be done and get an e-mail notifying you of a new incident of your name being found. Of course, the more common your name is, the more notices you will get about people other than you.

> **I used to be on our school basketball team. I hung out with my teammates whenever I had time. Then I broke my leg skiing and ever since I have had terrible pain. I thought it would end when the cast came off, but it has gotten worse. My doctor says the pain is complicated and has put me on the waiting list for a pain clinic. I can't play basketball anymore and it means I never see my friends. What can I do?**

It sounds like you had time with your friends off the court as well as at practices and games. Are you keeping yourself out of situations where you might see them because you no longer share the sport? Or are they avoiding you?

Either way, if these are the people you want to spend time with, why don't you go by the gym at the end of practice and see if they are available? You can explain that you are having ongoing problems from your broken leg but are hoping to be back on the team at some point. If there are things that make your leg hurt more (like standing for a long time), suggest doing an activity that helps you avoid it.

If someone says something like "Your leg looks fine. Is there really something wrong with it?" you can tell them that there has been some damage to the nerves in your leg and that you are waiting to get treatment.

I'm 17 and have cystic fibrosis. I have a problem with social networking. Don't get me wrong, I love Facebook. When I am in the hospital, it keeps me in touch with my friends. For the people I hardly see in person anyway, things can go on almost like normal. But there are some things I'm finding hard. I have to be in the hospital at least once a year, and usually for four to six weeks for bad infections. Every day I am reading about the great things my friends are doing, seeing pictures of them together, and I can feel really alone. My mom says that that I shouldn't look at this stuff, but it helps me feel more connected. I know this doesn't really make sense, but it is how I feel. Who is right, me or my mom?

Feeling opposite ways at the same time may not make sense, but it is part of how people are. Usually little kids don't experience this or aren't aware that it is happening, but at your age, it is totally normal.

It isn't physically possible to be in two places at once, but it can sometimes seem like you are, thanks to electronics: you are both in the hospital and with your friends somewhere in the cyber-universe. But keep in mind that you are not sharing their experiences but rather just their reporting of what is happening to them. While this is a lot better than being totally out of the loop, it still doesn't make up for face-to-face socializing.

Try to keep in mind also that while they are raving about all the great stuff that is happening, they probably are not writing about all the boring, regular life things that are going on. From afar, it looks like other people's lives are a constant stream of drama-filled moments. Remember, though, from when you weren't in the hospital how people's real and online lives differ.

Is there a way you can get some of your friends to visit you in the hospital? See if your parents will pay for pizza once a week for a group of your friends.

Although the hospital staff won't let you hang out with other teens with CF (because your weird germs may be different from their weird germs and they don't want you to infect each other), they may be able to introduce you to people with other conditions who are going to be in the hospital for a while. A teen lounge, if there is one in the hospital, is another place to meet people and participate in activities rather than lying in bed.

When my parents found out last year that I had HIV, they told me about it right away and said I had to be really careful not to give it to anyone. I don't want to tell anyone at school about it, but how do I explain that I can't trade food out of my lunch bag or tackle them when we play ball?

You don't have to explain any of these things. There are only two ways people can get HIV from you. One is to get some of your blood into their body. This could happen if, for example, you donated blood or if you were sharing needles while injecting drugs (like anabolic steroids or speed).

The other way is by having unprotected sex with someone. The virus can be in cells in your semen and get into your partner's body if you have penetrative sex (anal, vaginal or oral) without a condom.

You cannot give someone HIV by trading cookies, tackling them, hugging them, changing in the same dressing room, drinking from the same water fountain or any other such activities.

It would help you to get some more information about HIV. There may be other things you don't understand or are causing you anxiety that could be fixed by knowing more.

Someone at the clinic you go to should be able to explain HIV to you, or you can get some pamphlets from the clinic, any birth control clinic, or your local AIDS organization. This group may have a support group for people your age or may be able to "buddy" you with someone who can help you understand more about HIV.

I don't know what I am doing wrong. I don't seem to have many friends. When I am with a bunch of kids at school, I try to joke around and stuff, but it doesn't seem to work. I don't think it is because of my disability. What can I do to make friends?

When something isn't working, it is time to try something new.

Not everyone is going to want to be your friend. When you do find a group of people who you want to get to know, you have to know how to approach them and decide how to fit in with them.

Teens who haven't had as much chance to be around other people the same age (because of being in the hospital or spending more time at home) often have a hard time knowing how to act.

This difficulty is made worse because many teens have been brought up to think they shouldn't criticize people who are disabled or ill. If others were acting in a way that bothered them, they would just let them know they should stop it. They may not feel as comfortable telling you that they think you are acting goofy.

If you have a friend, talk with him or her about your problem. Ask your friend to honestly tell you if there are things you are doing (like joking around too much or talking too loudly) that are turning people off. You can even ask your friend to signal you if you are behaving in a way that might bother people.

You can watch other people together and see what they do. You may notice that people are often included when they show they are interested in a conversation by looking at the speaker (without staring at them), nodding their head every once in a while and smiling when something is funny. You may be spending so much of your energy worrying about how you are doing that you forget about the other people.

Don't be so interested in making friends that you will do anything for anyone who acts nice to you. If the price of getting into a group is doing things that you don't feel comfortable about, or putting up with being put down all the time, think about starting another search for new friends.

I seem to keep on losing friends because we get into fights. What can I do so that I don't fight with them?

Getting into arguments or fights with friends is normal. All friends fight sometimes. It may be that how you fight and the reaction you have to arguments are the real problem. Of course, you shouldn't be fighting all the time.

When you have a fight, do you assume that the friendship is over? Do you give the relationship another chance, or do you just move on? It may be that when you were younger, you didn't have as much chance to learn about this part of a relationship. Maybe you weren't around other kids very much, or some kids' parents told them they shouldn't fight with you because of your condition. Now that you have friends who are willing to have a full relationship with you, maybe you see fights as the end of a friendship instead of being part of the process of a friendship. It is OK to call a friend the next day to talk things over. If you think you went too far, you can apologize. If your feelings were hurt, make that clear too.

When you argue with a friend, you are learning to stand up for yourself. In an argument, you sometimes learn how you really feel about something. Or it can be a way to "try on" a belief or idea.

Here are some rules about arguing with friends:

1. Never make fun of them or their family.
2. Disagree with their ideas, not with who they are. (Say "That is a ridiculous thing to say" instead of "I can't believe you are so stupid.")
3. If you are yelling so much that your throat starts to hurt, call a time out.
4. Make sure you understand what they are saying before you disagree with it.
5. Try to keep an open mind.
6. People's feelings are always legitimate. Don't tell someone he or she isn't angry or sad or whatever.
7. If you are fighting about what to do (as opposed to what you believe), see if you can find a compromise that you can both agree on.

If all you do with friends is argue, consider the possibility that you are provoking arguments. You may even want to ask someone with whom you have argued in the past if he or she thinks you were always starting fights, or if you seemed unfair in the way you fought.

Having friends is very important. It can be hard to know how to handle a relationship. The clinic you go to may have a social worker or adolescent medicine doctor or nurse who can offer you some help in making and keeping friends. This is often referred to as "social skills training" and can be helpful. Then get all the practice you can.

I hang out with a group of friends. Some of them have known me for a long time, and although I never realized it before, my newer friends see how they act with me and do the same. Now, someone new has entered the group, and she is acting weird. She seems to think it is so awful that I have a disability and that I should be treated like a baby. I hate the way she acts. She thinks I can't (or shouldn't) do anything. She talks to me very slowly and carefully, using short words. She seems to think that she is doing some kind of good deed by being with me. How can I get her off my back?

It would probably be wise to talk with her. You can explain that she seems to think you are incapable of doing anything, but you know there's lots you can do. Let her know that you are able to ask for help if you need it, and that if you don't ask for help, she can assume you can manage on your own.

If you don't want to talk with her directly, you may want to ask a friend to talk with her. But be careful. She will now have the message that you can't talk for yourself.

If there is something you know you can do better than she can, you may want to make sure she knows about it. Show her your article in the school paper or some other accomplishment, or offer to help her with her math homework.

I am getting tired of people telling me how skinny I am. Girls at school will either say things like "I wish I had your disease, I'd love to be so thin" or they ask me if I have anorexia. What can I do about this? Also, do you have any tips for gaining weight?

What you are experiencing is very common and very annoying. Girls have been so brainwashed about the desirability of being thin that some are willing to starve themselves to be thin, and even imagine that it would be worth it to be sick. The weight that many girls think is ideal is, in fact, so low that it is unhealthy. There is little room for acceptance of the idea that we come in all shapes and sizes, and that our worth does not depend on our appearance.

Teens with chronic conditions can suffer both because of weight loss and because of weight gain. Many are at the high end of the weight spectrum because of medication or because they cannot get enough exercise. Many are at your end of things and are thin because they need more calories, have decreased appetite, feel nauseated or don't absorb food as well as healthy people.

It can be helpful to have a standard answer for people who say they wish they had your illness. You may want to pick the worst aspect and say, "I'd be happy to take your weight and give you my (two months of being in the hospital every year, constant pain in my knees, hair falling out…)" or just "I can't believe you want to change how you look! Your weight seems perfect." It usually isn't a good idea to point out to the person how rude he or she is being.

If your problem is that you don't absorb nutrients, talk to your doctor, who might have some suggestions, such as drinking an elemental supplement (it's kind of like baby formula). If nausea is the problem, your doctor may be able to prescribe something to help.

If your difficulty in gaining weight comes from low appetite, there are various things you can do. It may sound old-fashioned, but fresh air really does seem to stimulate appetite. Try to get outside every day, even if the weather isn't great.

If you have been feeling depressed, get some counseling. Depression is a big cause of appetite problems and isn't any fun to live with. It can be helped.

Try eating foods that are what we call "calorie dense." These are foods that have a lot of nutrition packed into a small helping. Anything that is high in fat is calorie dense, and this would include ice cream, french fries, pies and other junk foods. Try this milkshake: 1 cup (250 mL) milk (not skim), 2 scoops ice cream, 1 tablespoon (15 mL) vegetable oil, 1 tablespoon (15 mL) wheat germ, 2 tablespoons (30 mL) chocolate syrup, and 1 raw egg (leave out the egg if you live outside Canada—salmonella in eggs is a big problem in many other countries). You can also use nutritional supplements like Boost or Ensure instead of milk in this shake, or add a powdered meal replacement. It is a good idea to talk with a dietician to make sure that none of these things will be a problem with your medication or condition.

It may be easier for you to eat small amounts frequently instead of big meals. You can carry a bag of nuts, raisins and chocolate chips around with you and have some between classes, on the bus and after school. Snack while you study.

Increase your exercise. Although this may seem counterproductive because it uses energy (calories), it may increase your appetite. It will help you put on weight in a good balance between fat and muscle (you need both).

I get treatments at night. This means that I can't ever stay over at a friend's house, something I would like to be able to do. I know the treatments keep me out of the hospital, so I should be grateful, but I feel like I miss out on a lot of fun.

Whether your treatments are dialysis, tube feedings or medications, the result can be the same. Being able to sleep over at friends' is often an important way of socializing. Kids talk about all kinds of things in the dark that they would never mention in the daytime. If you are never present at sleepovers, you are not as much a part of the group. And, as you point out, they are fun.

Is there any way your schedule could be changed to allow for two or three nights out a month? For instance, maybe you could be dialyzed or tube fed for four hours before going, and four hours the next morning. Yes, it would take eight hours out of your weekend, but you could read, have a friend over, play computer games or even do homework during the treatment.

If the treatment is short, you might be able to go home for half an hour or so late in the evening and then go back to the sleepover. If you don't feel comfortable telling people why you have to leave, you could say you forgot something at home. Make sure it is something that your host can't lend you. If you use this excuse too often though, people will either catch on or think you are really scatterbrained.

If none of these things seem possible, talk to your doctor about it the next time you have an appointment. It may be that it would be safe for you to skip one night a month, or there may be an alternative therapy you could use during the day.

If your friends know about your condition and the treatment, it may be possible for you to have them over. You might have to leave them alone for a bit (with a video and popcorn?) while you get hooked up. Remember, most of the time the lights will be off.

Often people with metabolic conditions, like glycogen storage disorders, must have a steady drip (often through an NG tube) all night or there will be serious consequences. If this is the case for you, make the point to your parents that you won't be living with them forever and that it is time for you to find and practice strategies to be away from them overnight sometimes. I know of young people who have gone on camping trips or away with their class to another city with these conditions. If there is an association or foundation for your condition, you could suggest that your parents ask there to be linked up with parents who have older kids who have made the transition out of home and into the world, for ideas about how this can be done safely.

If, in the end, your parents still won't agree to sleepovers, you should remember there are other kids whose parents won't let them go to sleepovers, or who go to their cottage every weekend, or who have jobs in the evening and who still have active social lives. You can still have friends and have a good time without ever spending a night away from home.

4

School and Work

SCHOOL TAKES UP MORE TIME than anything in your life except sleep. Even if you miss school when you are in the hospital, you spend time worrying about it. School can present special problems to people with chronic conditions. These problems can include people's attitudes, access to the programs you want, making up for work you have missed due to illness and appointments, and effects of your condition on your ability to get your schoolwork done.

Many teens have jobs to earn money to help support their families, to get spending money or to gain experience to move along a career path. Having a chronic condition may pose challenges to getting a job and may have an impact on career planning.

> **I'm in Grade 11 and I need to start making some plans for the future. I want to go to college, but I'm not sure what my ultimate goal is. Obviously, it will have to be something that can fit with the physical limitations of my illness. I talked to a guidance counselor at school who didn't seem to think I needed to be making plans at this point. Is he right?**

No, he's not. Teens with a chronic illness can benefit greatly from starting to think about career plans even earlier than other adolescents.

Your guidance counselor might be having a hard time seeing past your disease to the person you are underneath. He may assume that you'll need to be supported by your parents or the state when you are an adult. He might think he is sparing your feelings by not pursuing the subject of career planning because such a discussion will involve discussing your limitations and prognosis.

You should consider seeing an occupational therapist (your doctor can recommend one). She will help you figure out some general ideas of what you are ultimately looking for in a career by asking you about your interests, your personal style of working, whether you like working with other people or on your own and so on. She might have you fill out some questionnaires. She will then suggest possible careers that could fit with your interests and abilities.

Think about these choices. You don't have to make a decision at this point. You may find that the ones of most interest to you share a common educational pathway, such as computer training, a science degree, a secretarial course, an arts degree, teacher's college or trade school.

When you have mapped out a general direction, it is time to return to your school guidance counselor for help in applying for and getting into the kind of program you have chosen. Make it clear that this is what you plan to pursue and that you assume he will help you with this. He will have information not only on available programs but also about such things as financial aid.

I've missed a lot of school in the past few years, and even though I've tried to keep up, I feel there is still much catching up to do. I'm just finishing Grade 10. I'm feeling quite a bit better and don't

expect to be hospitalized again, but I still have appointments with my family doctor, my specialist, the physiotherapist and others. What can I do so that I don't fall too far behind?

First, figure out which of the people you need to see has the most limited, inflexible schedule. This is the person you have to plan around. Usually this will be the specialist.

Next, find out what kind of schedule your school is using this year. If it is a six-day schedule, or some other variation that fluctuates every week, you'll have the hardest time planning, but it can be done. A semestered program has advantages and disadvantages. If you miss a couple of months, you lose only the semester, not the year. On the other hand, you have less time to catch up on missed work.

Plan your courses. Don't take an absolutely full load. You need at least one spare (study hall, or whatever they call it at your school) every day. This way when you miss school, you won't miss as many classes, and it gives you time to catch up on what you've missed. Go to the guidance office and find out when the schedules for the next school year will be available.

Now, think about when you would like to have appointments. It is often unrealistic to think that you can go to a morning appointment and be back at school in the afternoon. Although afternoon appointments will interfere with after-school activities, they usually work out better. If you choose afternoons, find out which afternoons your specialist sees patients. Put this together with the schedule of classes you want and see if you can plan to have at least one spare on that afternoon. Don't succumb to the temptation to miss your least favorite subject most often. If you have your choice of more than one afternoon, pick the one on which you don't have an after-school activity. Try not to choose Friday afternoons—you'll miss all the planning for the weekend with your friends.

Find out from your specialist how often you are likely to need to go in, and make appointments for the whole school year on your chosen afternoon. The secretary might take some convincing to book that far ahead, but be firm. Let her know you understand that there might have to be changes, but the only time you can see the specialist is (for example) Thursday afternoons.

Now you have to talk to your physiotherapist and other caregivers. Let them know you are available only on the afternoons you have chosen. If they are in the same building, or near where your specialist is, see if you can make appointments for the same days. Have appointments with whoever tends to be on time before appointments with someone who often keeps you waiting.

Send a memo (no, I'm not kidding!) to your principal and guidance counselor, with copies to your teachers (when you know which you'll have) with the dates of appointments. Tell them there might be changes, but you are trying to keep all appointments to specific afternoons.

This seems like (and is) a lot of work, but if you do it, you will cut back on the amount of school you are missing, and your teachers will feel more comfortable knowing when you will be absent.

When school starts in the fall, remind your teachers that you will sometimes be absent on X afternoon. Ask them if you can get assignments the day before, and try to work on these assignments while waiting to see your doctor. Ask a friend to take good notes on those days so you can copy them.

Clustering your appointments and being able to plan ahead should help you keep up. Your teachers are more likely to give you a hand with the work when they see you making this effort.

Last week I had a seizure at school. I have only one or two a year, and this is the first one I've had at this school since I started a year ago. Fortunately, my best friend was in the class and stopped some guy from sticking his pencil in my mouth so I wouldn't "swallow my tongue." She also told the other kids it was no big deal and not to worry. My friend says that the teacher fluttered around like she didn't know what to do. Now the teacher is being kind of gooey sweet and sympathetic to me. I think my classmates would forget the whole thing if she would act normal (or as normal as a teacher can be). Can I get her to stop without making her mad?

This shows why it can be important to have a friend who knows about your condition. She intervened for you, and in addition to preventing someone from doing something stupid, she provided a role model for the other kids in your class. Now they know they don't have to see this as a big deal, and if you do have a seizure again at school, there are a whole bunch of people who know what to do.

See if your local epilepsy association or your doctor has an information sheet that you can give your teacher to inform her about seizures and what to do if a student has one. Take it to her after school and tell her that you thought she might like more information. (Don't say that it is so she'll know what to do next time—she won't like it if you imply she didn't know what to do last time, even though she didn't.)

Acknowledge that she must worry you'll have another seizure in her class. Tell her you won't have a seizure from working too hard, having too much homework or being criticized if your work isn't up to expectations. Make sure she knows that she cannot cause you to have a seizure.

If you don't want to talk with her, ignore her preferential treatment without doing anything that would seem hurtful. She will almost certainly get tired of treating you differently from the other students after a while and will revert to her usual self.

You probably won't believe this, but the boys' washrooms at our school don't have doors on the stalls. One of the teachers says that it's because kids kick them down. My best friend says that the teachers are so paranoid that they think us boys will have sex in the washrooms if we have any privacy. Whatever the reason, it's a real drag for me. I have to catheterize myself every few hours and it isn't something I want anyone to see. Right now I go to the nurse's office, where there is a bathroom with a door, but it is pretty far away from some of my classes. I tend to put it off longer than I should because I don't want to be late.

You are going to have a hard time winning this one, I'm afraid, but I think you should try to get this situation changed. As far as I'm concerned, everyone has a right to some privacy, not just you. I'm willing to bet that the girls' washrooms have doors on the stalls.

Gather your information first. Write to the principal and ask for the official reason that there are no doors. You don't have to tell him why you want to know. If you don't get an answer within a couple of weeks, make an appointment to see him. If he tells you (either in person or in a letter) that it is because of vandalism, find out when this happened. Maybe it was five years ago, in which case few, if any, of the culprits are still at your school. Now prepare your arguments and put them into a letter. Again, you don't have to say why you want doors. If you don't mind putting it in, however, it might strengthen your position. Point out that it is your understanding that the girls have doors and therefore you are being discriminated against on the basis of sex. Put in whatever good ideas you have. Before making your final copy of the letter, ask one of your parents or a teacher whom you trust to take a look at it. You should get a reply within a month. If you don't, start pestering. If the school says it won't do anything about it, send a copy of your correspondence to your local school trustee.

If you don't have the patience to fight this out, maybe you can work around scheduling a bit. If you go to the nurse's office and catheterize right before school, can you wait until lunch? Ask your doctor if it is OK to catheterize both at the beginning and at the end of your lunch hour. If you can do this, then you might be all right until the end of school. If you have lunch at some ridiculous time like 11 o'clock or even first thing in the morning, like some of my patients, then the afternoon may be too long. If you have a study hall (or spare), perhaps you can change your schedule so that it is in the afternoon and use the bathroom then.

I use a couple of Internet-based programs for my schoolwork. They make a huge difference to me and I don't think I would be doing so well in school if I didn't have them. Even though they were initially suggested by a psychologist from the Board of Education, my school now says that no one can use the Internet in classes. There are some classes where it is available, but the teacher controls what sites can be accessed. I have a tablet that has Internet access, so I have been using that. But my teachers are catching on, and one

of them reported me. Our new principal says that even though I might be using it educationally, other students were abusing the "privilege" of being connected, and so to be fair, now no one can use it in class.

Principals often like the "unfair for all is fair for everyone" approach. I don't get it, myself.

I'm assuming that you have already explored downloading the programs or finding similar programs that aren't Internet based.

You might have what is called an IEP, an Individualized Education Plan. If you do, the Internet help you are getting is probably laid out in your IEP. If it is, then your school has to follow what it says. If there is a guidance counselor who deals with "special needs," go to him and ask to see your IEP. If you don't have one or if it doesn't specify the use of the online programs, then get in touch with the school board psychologist who suggested them in the first place. She will probably be pretty annoyed that her advice is being thrown out the window and will help resolve the situation.

I get tired easily, and as silly as it may seem, writing tends to tire me out. The more tired I get, the more of a mess my notes are. Several of my teachers actually collect our class notes and mark them every couple of weeks. I lose points for messy writing, "lack of organization" and missing information. Often, I just stop taking notes when I am worn out, so in addition to low marks on my notes, I don't have anything to study from.

You have two problems here. The first is the price you pay when your class notes are graded, the second is when you write tests and exams and are less prepared because you didn't have good notes to study from.

The first is one of the more ridiculous bits of educational philosophy I've heard of. It's hard to believe there are teachers who feel that the quality of handwriting in your notes is related to what you have learned in the class. It seems to me that people who, for instance, don't pay attention in class and therefore miss information will be penalized when they write the exam. What can you do when you are up against such pointless things as grading notes?

Try to find out if there is a school policy that notes should be graded. If this is the case, find out who is responsible for this policy. Go to this person and ask for the reasons for the policy. Perhaps you can suggest some alternative approaches. If notes are marked because there is concern that students are having difficulty organizing their thoughts, suggest that the school run a mini-course on how to take good notes. It is reasonable for a teacher to expect work that is handed in to be neat, but the purpose of class notes should be to help the student study. Students should not have to organize their notes to suit a teacher, but rather to fit their own style of studying. The policy of marking notes discriminates against students with learning problems, those who tire easily and anyone who does not think like a teacher.

If there is no policy, get together a group of students to approach individual teachers to ask them to stop this practice. Use the above arguments and any others you can think of.

If all this fails, your last option is to go to the principal or vice-principal and explain why you should be exempted from being graded on class notes. This is a last option because it does give at least the appearance of having an unfair advantage. Make it clear that it is important to you to attend school even when you aren't feeling perfect, and that you don't want to miss school when you are too tired to take notes. You may have to offer to hand in some other work to make up for this, but don't volunteer this unless you feel you have to.

The second difficulty is that your inability to take good notes when you are tired interferes with your ability to learn. If typing is less tiring for you than writing (and my opinion is that everyone should know how to type), perhaps you can take a laptop computer to class. But you'll have to weigh the energy savings of not writing against the energy expenditure of lugging it around from class to class, not to mention the expense. Another option is to record the classes. The disadvantage of this is the time required to listen to the recording. If you have a friend who takes good notes, he or she might let you photocopy them. Most libraries have a photocopy (remember to take lots of change with you). As the school year progresses, you will find that some of your teachers rarely say anything that isn't in the textbook. If you read in preparation for class, you will have less to write down. Make a note of what the teacher emphasizes, as it is more likely to show up on exams.

The most important thing is to listen in class. Some people are so busy taking notes that they don't actually absorb what they hear. No matter how tired you are, make an effort to look like you are listening and to ask intelligent questions. Teachers are human and are more kindly disposed to students who seem to be paying attention than to those who sleep, file their nails or look bored through class.

I'm so depressed. I used to be really good in school. I got almost all As and it didn't seem all that hard. It's not that I didn't have to study, but when I did study, it paid off. I also had interesting things to say. Then I was in a car accident. Everyone says I was lucky to survive. My best friend, who was driving, was killed. I was in a coma for a while and now they say that it's a miracle that I've done so well. But I don't feel like the same person. I study and study to get Bs. I was planning to be a doctor, but that's not going to happen now. It's hard to see any point in going on at this point, being stupid and dull and not having any potential.

I'm not going to say that you are lucky or that you haven't changed. You are a different person now, and your capabilities are different. I think it is way too soon to say that life isn't worth living, and I certainly don't think anyone should ever kill themselves because they aren't doing well in school.

You know that your ability to learn has been weakened by your head injury, but I'm not sure if you've figured out which of your capabilities didn't get hurt. I think it would be useful to find this out.

Why did you want to be a doctor? If it was because you are a compassionate person who really wants to help other people, then there are lots of other possibilities out there for you. If it was to make a lot of money, then there are other ways to do that (which also would involve much less education).

You need a good assessment with a psychologist who can do detailed testing on you that would help you figure out what is working well for you. This might even help you find alternative ways to study, ways that you could remember things more easily or figure things out. It might be that you can do better in school using some of these tricks.

It may be that assessments that you have had up until now have been done for your lawyer to show how bad things are, and by the insurance company to paint a rosy picture. Your interests will be better served by an assessment that isn't linked to any legal stuff.

You should also figure out what you want to get out of a career or job, through testing and conversations with the same psychologist or with an occupational therapist. It may very well be that you can get your needs satisfied in another career.

While you are working toward this, you need to tell your family doctor or pediatrician how depressed you are feeling. This is very common in people with brain injuries, and there are things they can do to help you.

I'm not blind, but I do have terrible eyesight. It gets worse when I am tired. I have a hard time doing my homework. If I make the font big enough to see easily, there are so few words on the screen, it stops making sense. It is also a strain to keep staring at a computer screen. It's easier for me to see things that aren't so close up. My mother has been reading me some of my schoolwork, but she is busy and I can't monopolize her every night.

I'm going to suggest that you monopolize the television instead. If you have a new-enough television, you should be able to connect your computer to your TV. Even if you use a tablet, this should be possible. You may need an HDMI connector, which is a bit pricey, but this will allow you to read in larger type, farther away. You may have to sit fairly close, but not as close as with your computer or tablet.

This will work better if you can touch-type, as it is hard to use it you have to keep looking from the keyboard to the TV and back again.

I've been having trouble with my schoolwork, mainly because I've missed a fair amount of school for doctors' appointments. Also, my teachers seem to think I have a bad attitude. I get detentions for being late to classes because I get tired and can't get around quickly. I don't go to the detentions. (Why should I? It's not my fault.) Now they are having some big conference about what to do about me. My mother is going to be there, and one of my teachers and the principal and someone from the school board. It drives me nuts that they are all going to sit around talking about me and I won't be there to defend myself.

Are you sure you can't attend? School personnel often feel uncomfortable when students go to conferences about themselves, but it is difficult for them to prevent your going, especially if you have your mother on your side. Talk to her and explain why you want to go. Ask her to get in touch with the person who will be chairing the meeting and explain that you are coming. She may need to argue a bit, but if she can stand firm, she is likely to be successful.

Don't go to the meeting without a plan. Write down what you think the problems are. Come up with solutions for each one. (This may include things the school should do differently and ways in which your behavior could change.) Make suggestions about how your teachers could help you keep up with your work. Indicate your willingness to follow through with extra work you may have to do.

How your teachers perceive your "attitude" has a big influence on how they treat you. If you had gone to the office and explained why you felt you shouldn't have to go to a detention, you might have helped them see you in a more favorable light. Go to this meeting with a positive attitude. Make sure they know you are there to help solve the problems. Make it clear that you don't feel you are the problem.

If they don't permit you to go to the meeting, put your view of the situation into a letter. Try not to accuse anyone of anything. Ask your mother to read the letter to the group and have her leave a copy of it to be included with the other notes from the meeting. Ask her to take notes and to discuss them with you when she gets home.

I am a 15-year-old boy and have been going to the hospital for two years because of back pain that started when I went down playing hockey and broke my tailbone. My life is a mess. My mom and I just got back from a meeting at the school— I'm failing everything. The principal and teachers know I am in pain, but they say that I should be in pain at school instead of at home. I miss so much school, and when I am there, my mind doesn't stay focused.

Chronic pain (that is, pain that goes on for a long time) is awful. No one can tell by looking at you that you are hurting and sometimes they just don't believe it. There are lots of reasons why school would end up being a problem for you.

To start with, I assume that you are on pain medications, and probably fairly strong ones. These can make it hard to concentrate and may also affect your memory of stuff you have learned. Your teachers might also give you a hard time because they think you are lazy, stoned or stupid.

Second, most people who have bad pain have difficulty falling asleep at night. If you are awake until four o'clock in the morning, you are going to have a hard time getting up before noon. It can then be hard to make yourself go to school for half a day. Maybe you can't even get there if you have to take a school bus.

Finally, after a while, it gets harder and harder to go to school. You are behind, you might feel out of the loop with your friends and going there just makes you feel worse.

I have a few suggestions for you:

1. If you aren't already going to a specialized pain clinic, this is a must. They will have a team of professionals (from medicine, nursing, psychology and other fields with lots of experience in helping young people with similar problems). There is likely to be a waiting list, but you will move up to the top of it eventually.

2. We know that feeling more relaxed and diverted can take your mind off the pain. You can learn deep breathing, and try focusing on a calming experience, like listening to your favorite music or watching TV or playing video games. Try to involve yourself in these activities, especially when you are in pain. Many people have found that mindfulness meditation is also helpful in dealing with pain. Your doctor might know about a free meditation course, which are sometimes offered through hospitals. Meditation will not make the pain go away, but it will help you focus your mind despite the pain.

3. Consider asking to do your schoolwork online while you are waiting for your pain clinic appointment. In general, I think young people are better off in school than out of it, but in your case it is just making you feel awful about yourself. Set a realistic schedule for yourself to do schoolwork every day, in whatever chunks of time you can manage.

4. Arrange to stay in touch with friends during this time. You are probably talking to them on Facebook, or maybe gaming with them. But it is also important to actually see people. When you are spending time with friends (talking or playing), this diverts your brain from paying as much attention to your pain. If there is a time of day that you feel a bit better, invite a couple of people over to watch a movie, play a game or just hang out.

I have a job after school at a fast-food chain. I have to run sometimes to get there, which makes me wheeze. Yesterday the manager came into the locker room and saw me using my puffer. She says I can't work there anymore if I have to take medication. She says it might affect my judgment or something. I need this job. Do I have any rights?

Yes and no. As a part-time employee, you have very little legal protection in most places. On the other hand, you have (in my opinion) a moral right to continue in your job.

Write the manager a letter. State how long you have been working there; if you have never called in sick to work, mention that. If you have been available on short notice to do extra shifts, point this out also. Tell her that huge numbers of adults and teens have asthma and hold down jobs without any problems. Make it clear that it is unfair for her to discriminate against you because of your condition. Ask your doctor to write a letter stating that your medications are safe and that you can work while using them. Include this with your letter.

Deliver the letter to her and let her know that you want an answer in writing. Send a copy to the personnel director of the chain (call the head office to get the name and address). Keep copies of anything you mail out or receive.

If you haven't heard back in a week, go back and ask her what is happening. If she can't give you an answer, call the head office. Call the Lung Association and let someone there know what is happening.

I would be surprised if you don't get your job back. However, if you aren't rehired, you may want to consider putting in a complaint to the Human Rights Commission or the equivalent where you live. Approach local media and try searching online for labor watch-groups, to put pressure on the chain to reconsider.

If it looks as though this will drag out a long time, start looking for another job so that you don't go too long without a paycheck.

I'm too short to get a drink from the water fountains at school. I get pretty thirsty. If I'm really desperate, I can stand on my toes and stick my tongue into the water, but I look pretty stupid doing it. Any ideas?

If you carry a backpack, there are a few options.

Carry a plastic cup (so it won't smash if you drop your pack) to school every day. Fill it at water fountains or in the bathroom when you want a drink.

Carry a water bottle. Fill it before you leave for school and refill it in the washroom.

If you are not alone in this (for example, if you can't reach, neither can someone in a wheelchair), ask the school to put a lower water fountain in a convenient place. It may be able to get special funding to do this.

I get terrible headaches almost every day. They often keep me awake at night. I try really hard in school, but sometimes I can't concentrate because it hurts so much. I don't have migraines and the medication my doctor has prescribed hasn't helped very much. I really want to get a job and make some money, but I'm worried that I won't be able to manage it.

Holding down a job when you are in pain can be very difficult. If you can use the work to distract you, it might help, but sometimes pain can be so bad that you can't be distracted from it. If you get fired because you miss work a lot, it could make it harder to get another job. I think you should deal with the pain first.

There are a few things you could do. One is to ask your family doctor to refer you to a headache or pain clinic. Tell her how the headaches are affecting your life. The clinic will work with you to figure out what is causing the headaches and will suggest different things you can try. It may be that meditation or biofeedback will work for you. The clinic should be able to give you advice about how to talk with your teachers about the pain and its effect on you, and some strategies for holding down a job when you have headaches.

I missed a lot of school this year because of being sick. Instead of doing a bit of everything, I put all my energy into two of my courses, and got As in them. I didn't even write the exams for the others. Now, the school says that if I want to be considered to be in Grade 10 next year, I have to make up two more courses in summer school. I don't think it really matters to me what grade I am in. Does it make a difference whether they call me a tenth grader or eleventh grader?

For a change, I am going to agree with your school. Unless you had some fabulous plans for the summer, you should take the courses. You'll still have free time, and the summer won't pass by without you. If you have a trip to Paris planned, then forget summer school (but see if you can get a French credit for going).

Many things that happen in high school are centered on what grade you are in. In subtle and not so subtle ways, you will be left out of the activities that many of your friends participate in. Without as many shared classes, you will have less opportunity to see them and not as much to talk about when you do. Weekend plans are often made in the halls between classes. If you aren't around, you might be left out. Unless you have friends who are a year behind you, you will be in classes with people you don't know—like going to a new school.

Your transcript would show that you repeated a year—not the best thing for getting into college or university.

Finally, summer school tends to be easier than the regular year, so you can probably get a better grade than you would during the school year.

I have been in special schools all my life but I am about to start at a regular high school. I'm excited and scared. Do you have any advice?

Be prepared! That's always good advice. Specifically, sit down and think about what your expectations are for this experience. If you picture yourself having hundreds of friends the first day and finding everything easy, then you will probably be disappointed. On the other hand, if you think it will be terrible, then you are setting yourself up for an awful experience. So you need realistic expectations and plans to deal with some of the more difficult aspects.

One of the big advantages of a regular school is that you'll have a chance to get to know a wide range of people. Some of these people may never have met anyone with your condition and might feel nervous about it. They may stare, ask stupid questions or even tease you. It is important to remember that they are feeling insecure and that is why they are acting like this.

One teen told me that when he went to a new school and had a tube in his nose (for feeding), he got lots of stares. People seemed to avoid him. The principal called an assembly and explained why he had the tube and that it didn't limit what he could do with other kids. Although he was really embarrassed, he found that the principal's talk helped. If you are the first person at your school with your condition, you may want to consider asking the principal to do this, or even allow you to explain some things about it. Even if you don't feel comfortable with this, let people know that you are open to questions. If someone is staring, you can say something like "Do I have food on my face?" or "Do I know you from somewhere?" or some other comeback. It forces the person to, in some small way, recognize that you are a person and not just something to be stared at.

If you have a friend who is going to the same school, ask him if you can hang around with him for a few days until you know your way around. It will help the other kids if they see you with someone they know.

Another advantage of the regular system is that it tends to be better academically. You will probably learn more. This may mean that you are behind where your classmates are when you start. You may want to get some special tutoring over the summer to help get ready. Be prepared to work hard. It may be a temptation to try to get out of doing some work on the basis of your condition. Do not give in to this temptation. If you do, you may have a feeling that you really couldn't have done the work, and you will feel bad about yourself. You will lose out on important educational opportunities. Consider asking a classmate if he will work on a project or assignment with you. Explain that your last school was somewhat behind in the work. This is also a good way to get to know other students.

I have been trying to get a summer job and have had very little luck. It is important, not just for the money but because it can lead to a full-time job after graduation. I have been honest about my condition. Is this why I'm not getting a job? I have made it clear that I can arrange doctors' appointments for when I am off.

I think you need to try to address potential employers' concerns. If you ask them when they call to say you don't have the job, they will say it has nothing to do with your condition.

You've started off well by addressing doctors' appointments, but I think you need to go further. Let them know your condition isn't contagious. Tell them you have thought about the job, and there is nothing your condition will interfere with.

If it will, be honest about that and suggest something that compensates (for example, "I type about five words a minute slower than my average classmate, but I make 10% fewer mistakes").

Tell a potential employer that research shows that "handicapped" employees have better-than-average safety records and that insurance costs will not go up.

If your condition isn't obvious, you may want to wait to mention it. If you have no special needs at the job, it may not be relevant. You can tell your boss when you've been working for a while and have shown yourself to be a good employee.

Your difficulty may or may not be related to your condition. Are you doing everything else right? You should be dressed appropriately for the interview: not grubby, but not overdressed either. Try to look calm, and don't fidget. Have names of people who will give references for you. Find out what the job entails before you go for the interview. If the job is with a company, find out what it does in general. If you know someone who works there, ask that person for advice. Don't ask what it pays until you are offered a job.

The kids at my school who seem interesting are all involved in the environmental club and the anti-racist group. I hear them arguing in the cafeteria, and I'd like to be able to join in, but I don't really understand what they are talking about. I am in special learning disabilities classes, and we never talk about that stuff. I can't read well enough to read the paper, so don't suggest that.

Your observation that political issues are interesting and exciting is certainly true. Teachers in both regular and special programs are often reluctant to discuss such issues because people tend to have strong feelings and disagreements about them. Special education teachers may also feel that kids in their classes would be unable to understand the issues.

Because the issues are often those of respect and fair treatment, I think you will be able to understand them, once you get some information.

There are now news programs on TV just for young people. See if you get one in your area, and try to watch it. They often give more background than adult news programs.

Ask your parents about issues. If one of them is in a union, he or she may be able to tell you something about labor history and some of the things unions are fighting for now.

Tell your social studies teacher that you want to hear about social issues in class. Ask her if she could explain a newspaper article once a week that has something to do with the environment, women's rights or equal rights for people with disabilities.

I am deaf and have always gone to school with kids who can hear. I lip-read and learned some sign last summer at camp. Ever since then, I have wanted to go to a school where all the kids are deaf. My parents have never wanted me to sign, but now they have agreed that I can go away to school. Now I'm worried about what it will be like.

Have you thought about seeing if you can go for a visit? You might be able to get a better idea of what to expect.

It is likely there will be things about it that you really like, and others that you won't.

You are going to get a chance to socialize with other kids in a different way than you have before. This may seem quite intense at first, and you may be able to prepare for it by learning more sign language. There are probably courses offered in your city. Even if you can't take a course, you will probably pick it up pretty quickly at school. It will be like a language-immersion course.

It is a big adjustment to move away from home. You will miss your family and friends. You may want to arrange to have someone you can talk with—a counselor or social worker.

Rules are very different at boarding schools than they are at home. It may take some time to get used to less independence. You will not have access to a car, curfews on weekends may be earlier than at home, and you may not have as much opportunity to just "hang out" at a local mall.

On the other hand, you will have the opportunity to learn sign and to have free communication in it with people your own age. You will become part of a community. You will be in a setting that is designed to help you learn.

Whenever people move, it takes about a year to adjust. Don't make any judgments too soon. Go for a year, see how you like it, then decide whether to return.

I got leukemia when I was 10. I missed a lot of school until I was 13. Since then (three years ago), I haven't needed any treatment and I don't miss much school. You'd think that three years would be long enough to catch up, but I find that I am still behind. I have trouble understanding assignments and getting organized. My mother thinks maybe she spoiled me when I was sick and so now I'm too lazy to learn. I feel like I work hard.

I doubt that you are lazy. If you were, you wouldn't be so worried about how you are doing in school. I don't think any of this is your fault or your mother's.

There are at least two possibilities here. One is that you missed very important, basic information when you were sick. It could be that you have learned facts and things since then, without having an underlying knowledge of its importance or how everything fits together. If this is so, you may need some help to go back and learn some basics. You could do this with after-school tutoring or summer school.

Many teens have difficulty with organizational skills. There may be courses offered in your community on how to get organized or a teacher at your school who could help you with this.

The other possibility is that this is an effect of radiation treatments to your head as part of your cancer treatment. In some people, this can cause long-term difficulties with learning or organization. If this is the case, it doesn't mean you can't learn, but it does mean that you will learn more easily with special help and teachers who know how to teach people with learning problems.

You should talk to a guidance counselor or psychologist at your school. Tell them about your concerns and ask to be tested to help find out why you are having difficulties at school. They should be able to make some suggestions about special programs or help.

Show your mother this section of this book. It sounds as though she is feeling guilty about all this, and it will be helpful for her to understand that it is not her fault.

There can by many "late effects" of cancer treatment that don't happen or become obvious until quite a bit of time has passed. When you go for appointments, the health care team should be addressing this with you. When you grow up, you will need to continue to have regular appointments to see if you are experiencing late effects. Many adult cancer centers have clinics for people who had leukemia or other cancers in childhood. Your current clinic should send you to one of those when you leave pediatric care. If they don't mention it, make sure you bring it up.

5

Alcohol, Drugs and Medications

TEENS WITH CHRONIC CONDITIONS are faced with conflicting messages about drugs. Your doctor and your parents encourage you to take your medications. Ads on TV tell you that drugs are bad. Some of the kids at school say that drugs are bad, but cigarettes and drinking are OK.

As someone with a chronic condition, you may have got a message that if there is something wrong, there is a pill to try to fix it. This is not the case. Most of life's problems cannot be solved through drugs. In addition, medications can interact with each other and with alcohol, cigarettes and street drugs.

You have probably already experienced unpleasant medication side effects. This chapter talks about some of the side effects that drive teens nuts and suggestions about how to deal with them. If you think you are having side effects, talk with your doctor. Never just stop taking your medication, unless you think you may be having a serious reaction (for example, difficulty breathing, major rash, agitation).

There is only a small amount of information available about alcohol, street drugs and chronic conditions. I have found what I can and have included it, either in answer to questions or in the charts at the back of the book, in Appendix 1.

My parents have never talked to me about alcohol. I think they assume that I wouldn't even consider drinking, since I'm on medication. I wouldn't mind being able to have a beer at a party every once in a while, but I don't want to do anything dangerous.

There are several factors you need to consider.

First is the chance of an interaction between your medication and alcohol. These could be such things as increasing or decreasing the effect of a drug you are on (either can be dangerous), increasing the side effects you experience, introducing new side effects and increasing the effects of alcohol. A disulfiram-type interaction is one where you get a bad headache, flushing, a racing heart, low blood pressure, nausea and vomiting when you drink while on a medication. Chart I in Appendix 1 lists some interactions of medication and alcohol. If your medication isn't mentioned there, or if you feel you don't have enough information, talk to your doctor. There are a number of medications that don't have a bad interaction with alcohol.

Second is the chance that alcohol will cause a temporary or permanent change in your condition. If you have a mobility or speech impairment, there is a good chance that it will get worse when you have been drinking. If you have any disease in your liver, drinking could result in long-term damage. Discuss this with your doctor.

Third, changes in your level of inhibitions and in your judgment while drinking could have a more harmful effect on you than on someone without a chronic condition. You might forget to take your medication. If you end up in an unsafe situation, you will be less able to escape or fight off an attacker. Teens who have had a head injury say that they can't control their behavior when they have been drinking and may do things that they regret afterward.

If you are going to drink, keep in mind that alcohol will make you pee more. If there is anything about your condition that requires that you to be well hydrated (like if you've had a kidney transplant), then drink at least the same volume of water as the beer or wine you are drinking. If you are drinking shots, then the amount of water you need to drink should be a lot more—6 to 8 ounces per shot.

All this sounds very gloomy. They are only possibilities. Everyone's situation is different. Look at the charts in Appendix 1. Think about all this. Discuss it with someone knowledgeable whom you trust, such as a nurse-practitioner or your doctor. These people know that teens drink and should have answers that are specific to your condition and medication.

I'm somewhat overweight and want to go on a diet. One of my medications always comes with a little sticker that says "Take with food." Will this be a problem?

It shouldn't be, because you shouldn't skip meals when trying to lose weight. Medications that are marked "Take with food" are usually irritating to your stomach if taken alone, especially if you make a habit of it. Other medications may need food in the stomach in order to be absorbed properly into your body.

Before you go on a diet, talk with your doctor or nurse-practitioner about your weight and see if she thinks it is necessary for you to lose some weight. You may be wishing for an unrealistically low (and unhealthy) weight.

If your doctor agrees that it is OK to lose some weight, take a close look at your life. Find out if any of your medications have contributed to your weight gain. If this is the case, it may be more of a challenge to lose the weight if you are still on the same dose.

How active are you? Teenagers who are overweight don't eat much more than their smaller friends, but they tend to exercise less. Do you watch a lot of TV? There is some evidence to suggest that you use less energy watching TV than reading a book. There is also a good chance that you snack while watching TV. No matter what your condition, there is some activity that is right for you—be it swimming (great for asthmatics), wheelchair basketball, walking or yoga. Be creative and find an exercise program that is safe and enjoyable.

If you are determined to diet, change your intake to a pattern that you can live with forever. Try to pick foods that are high in fiber and low in fat. Try not to eat a lot of white foods (white rice, white bread, french fries, and so on). Limit desserts to weekends. Avoid highly processed foods, the kinds of things that come already made. If you can replace chicken nuggets with a chicken breast or sandwich meats with tuna, you will be doing yourself a big favor. And don't skip meals, even if your medication is safe to take on an empty stomach.

I have been feeling lightheaded for a few weeks. It has interfered with my ability to concentrate at school, and my friends have said that I seem spacey. I went to my doctor yesterday and he said it was probably from a new medicine he started me on a month ago. Why didn't he warn me that I would feel this way?

There are few drugs that have only one effect. All effects except the one for which the drug is prescribed are considered to be side effects. (Side effects of a drug can therefore change depending on why someone takes the drug. An antihistamine taken for allergies can have the side effect of drowsiness. If the drug is taken to help someone sleep, then drowsiness would be the effect, not a side effect.) Most drugs have a long list of possible side effects, many of them uncommon.

If the side effect is not very common, the doctor may not remember to mention it. He may tell you about the things that many of his patients have experienced and about rare side effects that can cause big problems.

Some side effects are listed for almost every drug. Headache, nausea, diarrhea and rash are the most frequent side effects. It is hard to find a medication that does not list these as possible effects.

Some doctors do not warn patients about side effects because they know that when people know that they might have something like headaches or lightheadedness, they are more likely to get the side effect. When participating in research on medication, the patients taking a placebo (which looks like their medication but does not have any active ingredient) often experience the side effects they might expect to get on the real medication.

Other doctors minimize the possible effects of a medication because they are worried that patients will not take the drug if they know it has the potential to make them uncomfortable. There have been many teenaged girls who wouldn't take the birth control pill because they thought it would make them fat (pregnancy doesn't?), even though as many people lose weight on the pill as gain it.

I believe that people have a right to know about possible side effects and complications of any treatment. If this is important to you, let your doctor know that you want to be warned about side effects in the future. If he is reluctant to tell you, you might be able to get side effect information from your pharmacist, or on the Internet (look at the manufacturer's website) or at the public library.

Always call your doctor if you are on medication and experience severe shortness of breath, wheezing, blurred vision, loss of vision, numbness in any part of your body, rash, continued flushing (redness) of your skin or severe dizziness.

Never stop a medication because you think you have a side effect. Call your doctor first to discuss it. It may not be related to the drug, or it could be a side effect that is limited to the first few days of use.

Ever since I started on a new medication, my acne has got much worse. Could this be related or is it just a coincidence? Intellectually, I know it is better to have zits than to be sick but, to be honest, sometimes I think the zits are the worst thing that could happen to me.

It is tough when a medication changes your appearance for the worse (and I've never heard of a drug that turns people beautiful as a side effect). This is a big reason why teens skip their medications.

Acne can be caused by many drugs (see Chart A in Appendix 1), but even if you are on one of these drugs, it may be from something else.

There may be a solution to this problem. If the acne is from prednisone or another steroid, an antibiotic that you put on your face often works wonders. Talk to your doctor. She may want to send you to a dermatologist (skin specialist). It may be that starting an acne medication or changing to one that is stronger will improve the situation. Your doctor may be able to switch you to a different medication or change your dose of the one causing the problem. Any doctor who cares for teens should understand what a big problem this is for you. If you feel you are not being taken seriously (for example, if she says, "No one ever died from acne"), consider asking your family doctor or pediatrician to refer you to a skin specialist.

Whatever the solution, keep in mind that it won't work overnight. Continue with the plan for a few weeks to see if it is going to have an effect.

My face is getting so hairy that other kids are starting to notice. I've been going for electrolysis, which hurts and doesn't seem to make much difference. Other girls don't seem to have to deal with this. What could be causing this?

Hirsutism (the medical name for hairiness) can be caused by internal or external factors. That is, you may have a hormone imbalance within your body that results in more hair growth, or it could be from a medication you are on. Hairiness also tends to run in families.

It is important to see your doctor about this. Even if you are on one of the medications listed in Chart B in Appendix 1, this still could be a problem originating in your body. Before you go to the doctor, look at the other women in your family. If your mother has a lot of hair on her face, you could ask her when she first noticed it. Your doctor will probably ask you how hairy your female relatives are.

Your doctor will also ask you questions about your menstrual history and may want to take some blood.

If your doctor thinks this is due to your medication and switches you to something else, don't expect the hair to go away immediately. It can take months for the hairiness to resolve.

This is another area where it can help to have a snappy answer. I heard about a girl who, when asked why she has hair on her face, says, "I took it up as a hobby."

If you can't switch medications, you may just want to try bleaching the hair. You can use peroxide, which is fairly gentle. The hair will still be there, but it will be harder for people to see. Try it on a small part of your skin first, to make sure that your skin can tolerate the peroxide.

People who are on immunosuppressants (like prednisone, azathioprine, tacrolimus, cyclosporine, sirolimus and others) should not have electrolysis without first consulting their doctor or nurse-practitioner.

Never use products that remove hair from legs on your face. These creams are quite harsh and the skin on your face is not as tough as on your legs. Smelling them often makes people feel sick, so applying them so close to your nose could also be problematic.

I'm too embarrassed to talk to my doctor about this: I don't feel like having sex very much anymore. In fact, I hardly ever even think about it. Last week, when I tried to make love with my girlfriend, I couldn't get it up. How can I figure out what is causing this, and what can I do?

This may take some detective work on your part. There are many causes for a decrease in sexual desire (libido) and impotence (not being able to get an erection). Some of these are discussed in Chapter 6.

Charts C and D in Appendix 1 list medications that can affect sexual functioning. In addition to decreased libido and impotence, drugs can often interfere with ejaculation in men and orgasms in women.

Alcohol, marijuana and other drugs have been linked with the problems you are experiencing (see Chart H in Appendix 1). If you are using them, you should consider stopping completely for a month to see if there is any improvement. If there is, you will have to decide which you want more—to keep on getting drunk or stoned, or to have sex.

Some of the worst offenders are antihypertensive agents (drugs to reduce blood pressure) and cimetidine (for ulcers). Many teens with chronic conditions are on these medications.

Another group of drugs that cause sexual problems are SSRIs, used in treating depression and anxiety. In addition to problems with sexual desire and erections, they can also lead to difficulties in having an orgasm. The herbal remedy gingko biloba is sometimes recommended to counteract this effect. People who are on insulin or anticoagulants (blood thinners) shouldn't take gingko. There also have been reports of problems with liver function in people who use gingko. There is no research that proves that gingko works.

If, after thinking about the possibilities and looking at the charts in Appendix 1, you think your problem might be drug related, you should talk to your doctor. If none of your medications are listed on the charts, still go to your doctor, as I haven't listed drugs less commonly used with teens. I know it is hard to discuss these things, but the payoff could be big. Sometimes just a decrease in dosage can restore sexual function. It may be possible to substitute another drug. For example, ranitidine is similar to cimetidine in action but does not affect sexual function.

Explain to your girlfriend what is going on and ask her to be patient. She may be worrying that you don't find her attractive anymore. Once she is reassured, she may enjoy the chance to spend some non-sexual time with you, or to try sexual activities that don't require an erection.

I am a 17-year-old with cystic fibrosis. Last week I got drunk at a party, and the next day I felt terrible. Not only did I have a humungous hangover, I also coughed more than usual and my chest felt tight. This isn't the first time this has happened. I don't drink all that often, but I would like to be able to party. Do you think it was all the cigarette smoke at the party?

Many people with cystic fibrosis have reported what you describe, especially after drinking beer. A majority notice difficulty breathing and increased coughing even when they were not in a smoky environment the night before (although the smoke certainly doesn't help things). It seems that this effect is directly related to drinking. It may be that you sleep more heavily when you've been drinking and therefore don't clear your lungs by coughing. People also get a bit dehydrated when they drink, which may thicken secretions. In addition to respiratory complaints, some teens with CF who are on cephalosporin antibiotics get a severe reaction if they drink. They get a headache and they throw up. This happens soon after drinking.

At the next party, try drinking less than you did at the previous party, consider drinking something other than beer and drink lots of water. Don't drink when you are taking cephalosporin antibiotics (they tend to have names that start with "kef" or "cef."

In case you are thinking of switching to marijuana, I should warn you that increased congestion and coughing can also be associated with smoking marijuana. Many people with CF find that if they smoke marijuana, their symptoms improve for a short time but then get worse.

When my friends get sick they can just go to the drugstore and get something to take. They don't go through the hassle of getting a prescription, waiting to get it filled and paying a ton of money. If I get a cold or something, can I do this too?

Medications that you can buy without a prescription are called over-the-counter (OTC) drugs. It is not always clear why some drugs require a prescription and others don't. There are some countries where most drugs are OTCs and some countries that have much stricter rules.

OTCs can have many side effects and can interact with other drugs in the same way that prescription medications can. For example, they may reduce the levels of your prescription medication, leading to a decreased effect. Or you can have increased levels, leading to side effects. Some foods can even interact with drugs. I've included licorice on the list, as it is sometimes found in cough drops or cough syrups. Also, some OTCs may be more problematic for patients who already have certain conditions, such as high blood pressure or diabetes (high blood sugars).

Chart G in Appendix 1 describes some OTC prescription interactions, but there can be many more. It is unwise to take any medication without first asking your doctor. Some OTCs don't work anyway, so at least some of the time your friends are just wasting their money.

I had never thought of cigarettes as being a drug before, but someone said something to me the other day that made me think they are. I don't want the big no-smoking lecture. Just tell me if my smoking will have any effect on my medications.

You are right in suspecting that smoking can have an effect on levels of some drugs. It is thought that most of these interactions result from things called polycyclic aromatic hydrocarbons, which stimulate the liver and can reduce blood levels of a number of medications. Nicotine (the stuff you're actually addicted to) can also be involved in adverse interactions.

These problems can continue for several months after you quit smoking. The more you smoke, the more likely you are to run into trouble. Chart J in Appendix 1 lists some possible interactions. If you are on any of these medications, think about asking your doctor to check your blood levels, if that is possible for the meds you are taking. If you decrease your level of smoking or even quit, you may need less medication after a few months, so again, see your doctor for your blood levels.

Some drugs that do not seem to be affected by smoking are codeine, phenytoin, warfarin and steroids.

I'm sure my parents smoked marijuana when they were younger, but they give me these talks about how I shouldn't smoke dope—my grades will instantly plummet, I'll turn into a zombie and it will combine with my medication to make my skin turn green. I'm sure the first two won't happen, but I do wonder about the last one. Not that I think I'll actually turn green, but could it affect my reaction to medication?

Interactions between marijuana and some medications have been documented. Chart K in Appendix 1 shows the available information. There aren't a lot of medications on this chart, not because we know they're safe, but because the available literature is fairly small. Researchers certainly wouldn't get a bunch of teenagers stoned and then check their medication levels!

Because of this, you should know that you are taking a risk if you smoke up while on medication. I'm not going to give you a big harangue about how you shouldn't do drugs (although I will point out that you don't have to smoke marijuana just because your parents did), but it is important that you understand this may be a risky thing to do. If you do decide to smoke marijuana, make sure that someone you are with knows you take a medication. Be in a place where there is a telephone, in case there is an emergency. If your condition seems to be worse in the week after, consider getting your blood levels of your medication checked.

Marijuana is often contaminated with fungal spores. Teens who are taking high doses of medicines to weaken their immune systems (immune suppressants) have a chance of getting a fungal infection from smoking marijuana. This isn't common, but it is a gross way to die, so I thought I would mention it.

No one knows I do coke sometimes. My parents and my doctor would kill me if they found out. I could never explain to them how much it helps me cope with all the garbage I have to put up with because of my condition. I wonder about what it might do, whether it is bad to combine it with my medication, or if it will make my disease worse.

There are some significant problems associated with repeated cocaine use, many of which I'm sure you've heard about. If you have heart disease or high blood pressure, you are taking a huge risk, as cocaine has been shown to cause heart attacks, irregular heart rhythms, high blood pressure and inflammation of the heart even in people with no previous heart problems.

As with marijuana, there has been little published about interactions between cocaine and medications in humans. It is unclear whether animal studies are relevant. I could not even find enough information to make a chart for Appendix 1.

The combination of alcohol and cocaine has been associated with headaches, irritability, memory loss, possible liver damage, increased heart rate and sudden death.

Although it may seem helpful in the short term, it is impossible that using cocaine will help solve any of your problems. I don't think you are going to stop using it because of some possible dangers (as a colleague of mine says, "'Just Say No' just doesn't work"). Consider looking for some other ways of getting rid of the "garbage" in your life. It may be that you are depressed and that this is affecting how you feel about your condition and other issues in your life. Find a counselor you can be honest with, who will respect your right to confidentiality and who won't expect you to just give up drugs before you find some real solutions to your problems. Listening to you, I worry that you may be feeling like killing yourself. If the only solution you have been able to come up with is using cocaine, then I think you are probably pretty desperate. Get help now, please. (Just Say Help?)

I don't want to take drugs. I worry about the effect it may have on my condition or my medication. What do I do when someone offers me a joint at a party?

The easiest things are answers like "Not tonight, thanks" or "I'm the designated driver." Don't get into an argument about whether it is wrong to take drugs.

If someone is being pushy, you can always say, "I'm on more drugs than anyone in this room. I don't need to smoke too."

If you have friends who don't want to do drugs, try to go to parties and events with them. You won't feel that you are the only person in the world who isn't getting stoned, and it will give you some support.

It would be unrealistic to suggest that you leave any party where there are drugs or alcohol, as they turn up almost anywhere. But you need to be aware of the general atmosphere of the party. If you are feeling uncomfortable with what is going on, trust your feelings and leave.

I am planning to go on the birth control pill and am starting to wonder whether it will work as well as it should, since I am on other medication. I can't talk to my specialist about this, as he always sees me with my parents in the room. Do you have any information?

Oral contraceptives can interact with a variety of medications. This can affect not just the effectiveness of the birth control pill but also the other medications you are taking. Chart F in Appendix 1 lists some of these interactions. What it doesn't address are multiple interactions. Very little is known about combinations of three or more drugs.

Only a few people will actually have the effect listed. For instance, not everyone who is on both the pill and carbamazepine will get pregnant. However, information in Chart F should help you decide whether the birth control pill is a good option for you. If you are going to be on a medication for a limited time and it's one that can decrease the effectiveness of the pill, you should want to add another method (such as condoms and foam) while you are taking the medication and until you finish that pack of birth control pills.

If you are old enough to be having sex, you are old enough to see your doctor by yourself, at least some of the time. Let your parents know that it is time you took more responsibility for your condition and ask to see your specialist by yourself. You don't have to bring up the subject of birth control the first time, but he should know fairly soon after you start the pill (or even better, before you do) because of possible effects on your illness, medications and lab values. For more about birth control and specific illnesses, see Chapter 6.

**The last time my doctor gave me a new prescrip-
tion he asked me how much I exercise. I didn't do
much then, and told him so. Now I want to do more
and I wonder if I should stop taking the medication.**

No, don't stop taking your drug. The first thing to do is to call
your doctor and find out if there might be a problem and what
you can do about it.

There are some interactions between exercise and medications. Exercise may help your condition, so you may need less
medicine. Some drugs may have increased side effects when
you exercise. Some common ones include:

Fatigue while on blood pressure medications, antibiotics,
antidepressants, anti-inflammatory agents, heart medications
(alpha- and beta-blockers) and chemotherapy.

Irregular heartbeat when taking tricyclic antidepressants
(not often used in teens for depression, but you may be on
these for sleep problems or to help with bed-wetting), antihistamines or beta-blockers.

Lightheadedness when exercising and taking antidepressants, antihistamines, beta-blockers, diuretics, sleeping pills or
tranquilizers.

Tendency to get overheated when taking antibiotics, antidepressants, antihistamines, beta-blockers, chemotherapy, de-
congestants, diuretics or tranquilizers.

This does not mean you have to stop exercising or stop
your medications. You may find that it helps to take breaks
more frequently, wear lighter clothes when exercising, make
sure you get plenty to drink and, if you are taking diuretics, eat
more bananas or drink tomato juice.

I go to two different specialists and have a family doctor. I am on several medications and I worry about taking them together. Sometimes I feel like a walking chemistry experiment. I hope I don't explode one of these days.

I don't think you have to worry about exploding. But there are some other possible problems with taking multiple medications to keep in mind.

It is unlikely that taking your medications at the same time will lead to a problem. However, get all your medications at the same pharmacy, or if this isn't possible, make sure that each pharmacist knows about the other drugs you are taking. Pharmacists often have computer programs that warn of any difficulties you may have if taking these drugs together.

Because any one drug you take has more than one effect on your body, interactions between drugs can be quite complex. Drugs taken together may have no significant effect on one another. One may increase or decrease the activity of the other. It can affect how the drug is processed and eliminated from your body.

One of the biggest risk categories for adverse drug interactions (bad things that happen when taking two or more drugs) is being elderly. If you fit into this category, you're reading the wrong book. Another risk occurs when more than one person is prescribing, especially if they are unaware of your other medications. If your body is unable to effectively process drugs because of liver or kidney disease, you are also more likely to have an adverse interaction. Finally, there are probably some people who have an inborn tendency to have interactions.

What can you do? Make sure all your doctors and pharmacists are up-to-date on what you are taking. Carry a list of your medications with you at all times (you can print off a list from MyMedSchedule or make a MyHealth Passport—see the Resources section, in Appendix 2). Don't take any over-the-counter drugs (medications you can get without a prescription) without first checking with your family doctor or pharmacist. Remember that alcohol, marijuana and other street drugs can also interact with your medication.

Here are some common interactions for specific condtions (listed alphabetically):

Allergies: Antihistamines can hide the side effects (such as ringing in your ears) of taking too much ASA (aspirin). Antihistamines will add to the effects of diazepam, narcotics, some seizure medications and muscle relaxants. It may be more dangerous for you to drive or operate other machinery. You may have difficulty concentrating in class and be sleepier than usual.

Anemia: Iron supplements can bind other drugs in your gut and carry them out of your system. Levels of tetracycline, doxycycline (used for some sexually transmitted diseases) and penicillamine (for arthritis) can be greatly reduced when taken with iron. Acetaminophen, captopril, folic acid and thyroxine can also be decreased.

Asthma: The advent of inhaled medication has reduced drug interactions for asthmatics. Cromolyn has only local effects. Although some inhaled steroid does get into your bloodstream, the amounts are low and unlikely to cause adverse interactions.

If you are diabetic, inhaled bronchodilators may increase your insulin requirement. They may also make high blood pressure medication less effective.

Theophylline levels in the blood can be increased, even to dangerous levels if taken with the enzyme inhibitors. Levels can be decreased, making the drug less effective, by enzyme inducers (some are listed in the Seizures description below) and increased by enzyme inhibitors.

Ketotifen can increase the effects of sedatives, antihistamines and alcohol.

Arthritis: The non-steroidal anti-inflammatory drugs (used frequently for arthritis) can decrease your body's response to blood pressure medication and diuretics. They can increase your risk of bleeding if you are on anticoagulants.

The usefulness of steroids can be reduced when taken along with carbamazepine, or phenytoin, both of which are seizure medications. This has also been reported as an issue with birth control pills, but I haven't observed this myself.

If you are on steroids or other medicines that weaken your immune system, vaccines may not "take" as well, so your health care practitioner might suggest repeating them when you are off steroids.

Methotrexate levels may get too high when used with ASA, non-steroidal anti-inflammatory drugs or some antibiotics.

Heart Disease: The anticoagulant (blood thinner) warfarin can have its activity reduced by cimetidine, cotrimoxazole and metronidazole. This could lead to a blood clot. It can have its activity increased by ASA and enzyme inducers, leading to bleeding problems.

Cholestyramine and colestipol, which are taken to reduce cholesterol levels, can bind other drugs to them so they stay in your gut and don't get absorbed into your bloodstream. Antacids and drugs to stop diarrhea also bind heart drugs. Digoxin, diuretics and warfarin can all be affected and shouldn't be taken at the same time. If you are on one of these binding agents and thyroid hormone (thyroxine), you should wait a long time between taking them.

Digoxin toxicity (resulting in nausea, vomiting, fatigue, headache and abdominal pain) can result from low potassium in your blood. This can occur when you take furosemide or hydrochlorothiazide. Symptoms may worsen if you are also on steroids. Verapamil can also lead to high levels of digoxin. Trimethoprim (an antibiotic that is either used on its own or in combination with another antibiotic called sulfamethoxazole) can also increase digoxin levels, although this is more common in elderly people.

High Blood Pressure: Non-steroidal anti-inflammatory agents (which you might take for menstrual cramps, headaches and joint and muscle problems) can decrease the effects of many drugs used to decrease blood pressure, including captopril. This is also true of ASA.

Verapamil can lead to increases in the levels of medications that are metabolized in the liver (such as phenytoin and theophylline). If taken with enzyme inducers (see Seizures section, below), its effectiveness may be reduced.

Propranolol can make asthma worse and decrease the effectiveness of inhaled bronchodilators.

Lupus: The usefulness of steroids can be reduced when taken along with carbamazepine or phenytoin, both seizure medications. This problem has also been reported with the birth control pill, but I haven't actually had a patient on steroids who has gotten sicker after going on the pill.

If you are on steroids or other medicines that weaken your immune system (immunosuppressants), vaccines may not "take" as well. This doesn't mean you shouldn't have your immunizations, just that you might need to have them repeated when you are off the steroids.

Methotrexate levels may get too high when used with ASA, non-steroidal anti-inflammatory drugs or some antibiotics.

Seizures: Many anticonvulsants have the property of making the liver work at a higher rate (these medicines are called enzyme inducers). Because of this, other medications may not be as effective. I once treated a girl who was pregnant for the second time, even though she was on the birth control pill and took it every day. She was also taking carbamazepine for her seizures. She didn't think she needed to tell her neurologist about the Pill, and the people in the clinic where she got birth control didn't know she was taking anticonvulsants.

Carbamazepine, phenytoin (Dilantin) and barbiturates can all lead to decreased levels of steroids, antidepressants, theophylline, antibiotics, warfarin and estrogen (found in birth control pills). Carbamazepine even leads to reductions in its own levels, so that increased dosages may be needed after taking it for a while.

Carbamazepine and phenytoin levels can be increased by enzyme inhibitors such as erythromycin, clarithromycin, cimetidine, fluoxetine, isoniazid and verapamil. You could then have symptoms of too much anticonvulsant (dizziness, staggering gait, sleepiness, double vision).

Ulcers: Antacids (those thick, white medicines that you seem to have to drink gallons of) can bind drugs so they can't be absorbed. They have a big effect on some antibiotics. Iron supplements are not absorbed well in the presence of antacids. Propranolol, diazepam, ASA and cimetidine may also be affected.

Cimetidine is an enzyme inhibitor and thus increases blood levels of a variety of medications, including theophylline, phenytoin, antidepressants and warfarin.

Urinary Tract Abnormalities: You may be on antibiotics to prevent infections or may have to be treated for frequent infections.

Trimethoprim-sulfamethoxazole (also known as cotrimoxazole) can make the body more sensitive to the effects of warfarin. It can increase phenytoin levels.

Erythromycin can increase blood levels of carbamazepine, tacrolimus, cyclosporine, sirolimus and theophylline.

Ciprofloxacin can increase levels of caffeine and theophylline.

Transplantation: Cyclosporine, tacrolimus and sirolimus can interact with a variety of medications. Levels are decreased by phenytoin, phenobarbital, carbamazepine and rifampicin. Cyclosporine, tacrolimus and sirolimus levels can be increased by oral contraceptives, amiodarone, azithromycin, ciprofloxacin, clarithromycin, clonidine, pulse steroids, erythromycin, fluvoxamine, itraconazole, ketoconazole, voriconazole and fluconazole, and also by grapefruit juice. When cyclosporine and cimetidine are taken together, there may be some changes in kidney function. Also, some over-the-counter medications (OTCs, or medications you can buy without a prescription) can affect cyclosporine, tacrolimus and sirolimus levels. Talk to your doctor, nurse-practitioner or pharmacist before taking any of these.

6 Sexuality

SEX. IT CAN BE HARD TO ADMIT that you have questions about it. I admire the teens I spoke with while writing this book who found the courage to ask questions about sex. Sometimes even identifying what your questions are can be hard and figuring out where to get answers can be a challenge. It is not surprising that this is the longest chapter in the book. I have tried to include all the information I could find about the impact of chronic conditions on sexuality, birth control and pregnancy. There is also some information about sexual development.

Remember as you read this that many of the questions you will have will have answers that vary from one person to another, and from time to time in your life. Only you can decide what is right for you. Just because your best friend is having sex does not mean you have to. Various family members may have different ideas about things like masturbation. Get the basic information that you need and then think about the issues involved. Make your own choices.

> **I am a 15-year-old with cystic fibrosis. I am quite small for my age and haven't started having periods yet. I feel that I get treated like a 12-year-old. Is there anything I can do to make my body grow up? Although I have lots of friends, no one ever asks me out. A couple of guys I've been interested in don't seem to have even noticed that I'm female.**

You share this problem with many young people with cystic fibrosis and with other chronic illnesses. With many conditions (such as CF and inflammatory bowel disease), growth delay and slowness in physical maturation are often a result of problems with diet, usually not getting enough calories (both because you need more calories and because you don't absorb nutrients well). With some illnesses, problems with growth are a side effect of medications like steroids. And with others, puberty is later than average because of the effects the disease has on hormone regulation. Teens who don't have CF or IBD and who aren't on steroids should ask their doctor why their development isn't at the same stage as their friends'. If it is due to their condition, the doctor should be able to give them some idea of when things might start happening.

If your physician or other health care practitioners have suggested that you limit your food intake, talk with them about your concerns about growth. Most CF experts are now advising a free diet, with no restrictions. Research still continues in the area of diet and bowel disease, but at this point many physicians also suggest that their patients eat what they want. Sometimes doctors will suggest nighttime tube feedings if you can't eat enough during the day.

See a dietitian for advice about how you can increase the amount of energy in your diet. She will be able to recommend calorie-dense foods—those that have more calories packed into them than average.

Remember that it takes time to grow and you won't see changes overnight. It might take your friends and classmates time to notice the changes too. The growth and development you experience will likely increase your self-confidence, making it easier to relate in a different way than as "just" a friend.

I'm 13 and I'm getting breasts. I'm a guy! Why is this happening? Am I turning into a girl? Is it from my medications?

You are definitely not turning into a girl. There are several possibilities.

The most likely is that you are experiencing gynecomastia of puberty, that is, breast enlargement in boys associated with the hormonal changes your body is going through. This is quite common. Studies differ, but from what I've seen, I would suggest that 10% to 25% of boys experience gynecomastia in puberty. This means that you are not the only guy in your gym class to whom this is happening. It is a condition that goes away by itself.

There are some conditions that are associated with gynecomastia. If you have liver disease, kidney problems (especially if you're on dialysis), poorly controlled hyperthyroidism or are recovering from malnutrition, you are much more likely to have gynecomastia.

Gynecomastia may be associated with ongoing use of alcohol, speed, heroin or marijuana. Gynecomastia can also be a side effect of medication. (See Chart G in Appendix 1.)

Because you are more likely to have a medical reason for your gynecomastia than someone who does not take medication or has a chronic condition, you should see your doctor about this. Chances are, though, that this is another sign of puberty, and one that will pass.

I've been talking to this girl I met online. She gave me her phone number and we have been texting each other. I sent her a picture of myself and she sent one back. Then the next day she texted me a picture of her with no shirt on, just a bra!

It was pretty exciting, but I felt a bit uncomfortable too, because I don't think I'm ready to send anything that revealing of myself (and my scars). I told a friend of mine, who asked to see the pic, so I showed it to him. Then he asked me to text it to him. He says that she sent it to me without me asking for it, so she probably won't mind other people having it too. I guess he has a point—do you think I should send it to him?

Even with all of the bad (and even tragic) things that have happened to people because of sexting (someone texting photos of themselves undressed, masturbating, etc.), it is still going on. Often, the story is put in terms of guys pushing girls to do this, but in my experience, it is just as common for someone to hear about it and think it is expected or a good thing to try. Once you have sent something like that, you don't have any control over it, and people have ended up with these photos all over the Internet and with everyone at their school seeing them.

Just because the girl didn't take this into account when naively sending you the photo doesn't mean it is OK for you to send it to your friend, who will send it to others. Depending on how honest you feel you can be with her, you might consider telling her why it wasn't such a good idea, despite your enjoyment of the picture. If she says something like "I knew I could trust you," remind her that she has never even met you.

I had radiation treatment when I was 12 and my right breast never really grew. I wear a sock in my bra, which looks more realistic than you might think, and I've never told anyone, not even my best friend. Pretty soon my boyfriend is going to discover it, unless I break up with him. I'm worried about how he'll react.

Unless you are planning a career as a nun, breaking up with him will postpone the problem but will not solve it. If you are happy with him and the direction your relationship is taking, now may be the time to address it. Leaving him to "discover" it is not a good idea. He is sure to be surprised, and your feelings may be hurt by his reaction.

I think you should talk to him about it before that happens. Tell him about the radiation and the effect it had. Let him know whether you want to be touched on the right side, and if you have the same level of feeling on each side. Make sure he knows that you haven't told anyone else and that it is private information.

Many guys are very into breasts, but that doesn't mean that he won't like both of yours. When you tell him about the different sizes, hopefully he will focus on the fact that he's actually going to be touching and seeing your breasts. I can't promise a good outcome, but if he has some advance notice, chances are things will go well.

I am a 17-year-old with lupus. I have been going out with this really great guy for a while, but I find that my sex drive is much lower than his. We enjoy our time together, doing lots of other things, but I hardly ever feel like having sex. When we do, I really like it, so it's not that.

There are a number of factors that could be involved, not all of which are related to your condition.

Many times, in otherwise happy relationships, there is a difference in sex drives. People do not all have the same need for sexual gratification. As well, there are differences in the time of day when people are interested in sex. Maybe you are a person who would rather make love earlier in the day, and he's an after-midnight type.

There may be things that unconsciously are worrying you about having sex. You might not feel completely ready for this experience. Maybe you feel nervous about not having enough privacy. If you are female, worries about pregnancy might be interfering with desire.

Depression can also interfere with sexual desire. You may want to examine how you have been feeling lately. If you think you've been depressed, talk to a health care provider about it.

Many people with lupus (and other chronic conditions) get tired easily and may be too fatigued to be interested in sex. If you feel you are ready to have a sexual relationship and have made plans to prevent pregnancy and sexually transmitted infections, you might want to make plans to get around fatigue. Have a nap before you go out. Consider planning in advance to have sex, and make it a time of day when you have more energy. You may want to have sex at the beginning of a date, then have a nap together before going out. Don't plan a bunch of other activities for the same day. Experiment with ways of getting sexually excited that don't take a great deal of energy (like talking about sex, or having him massage you).

Your medication may be suppressing your sex drive. Appendix 1 lists drugs that may have this as a side effect. You could consider talking with your doctor about changing medications, but there may not be a good alternative medication for you.

Your boyfriend may be feeling that it is his fault you aren't as interested in sex as he is. It will help him if he understands that this is a side effect of your illness or treatment, rather than a reflection of your feelings for him.

When I started high school I knew that I wasn't ready to get involved in a relationship. I noticed that dating and having a boyfriend or girlfriend

didn't seem to be a big deal at my school—in fact, the kids who are in a relationship are considered to be a bit odd. But now there is a lot of talk about people "hooking up." My friends don't talk about doing it themselves, but there are lots of rumors about other kids hooking up. What does this mean? Are they having sex?

The essence of hooking up is that it is a sexual interaction with someone who isn't in a relationship with you. People use the term in many ways—it can include kissing, touching each other and oral, anal or vaginal sex. Some teens may say that they hooked up when all they did was talk about having sex. These may be one-time encounters with someone you meet online, at the mall or through a friend. Sometimes people hook up more than once, but it doesn't usually turn into a relationship. Hooking up seems to be more common these days, although statistics show that teens are actually delaying having intercourse, and the percentage of teens having intercourse hasn't changed.

Why do people hook up? Sometimes they are curious about sex—they want to see what it is like but aren't in a relationship. They often want to avoid the emotional aspects of sex and just concentrate on the physical.

As I mentioned, by definition, when you are hooking up, the other person isn't in a long term relationship with you. They don't have as much incentive to tell you if they have a sexually transmitted infection or to try to be a great lover or even to think about your needs at all. Some kids say they like it for this reason, that they just get their own needs met and don't have to worry about someone else's. But these encounters don't always leave people feeling happy. Some kids tell me that they feel kind of empty after hooking up.

You could have a hard time tracking the person down if you end up with a sexually transmitted infection (or realize you might have given them one) or if you get pregnant. Someone might think that once you have agreed to the hook up, you can't change your mind, even if you get a creepy feeling or they just don't attract you. If you get sexually assaulted (including being forced into particular sex acts that the other person thought were part of the deal), you may find it hard to tell the police because you feel you agreed to it. The police may have a hard time catching the person, as they won't always tell you their real name.

You've noticed that there seems to be a lot of hooking up happening at your school, but that no one seems to be admitting that they are doing it. People often hook up with people outside their school because they are hoping to get into a relationship at some point and don't want a prospective partner to be scared off by knowing that they've had sex with a bunch of people. Also, many people who say they are hooking up aren't actually doing it. Instead, they are hoping to impress someone, are trying to hide that they are gay, don't know what it means or are saying it because they have heard other people say it.

I have a really good friend who is a guy (I'm a girl). He is one of the people who stood by me when I got sick and was in the hospital. Going back to school was much easier because he was there. He has suggested that we become "friends with benefits." Neither of us feels ready for a relationship, but both of us find that we think about sex and imagine it often. This seems like it might be a good solution. What do you think?

As you have implied, being "friends with benefits" means not being in a romantic relationship with each other but having sex. Teens have told me that they like this because they get their sexual needs met without feeling entangled. They can ask for what they want and demand safe sex without worrying that they will lose their boyfriend or girlfriend by being too assertive. One of my patients told me that she likes having a friend with benefits because if she had sex with someone she loved, she would probably do anything he wanted, even if she didn't feel comfortable with it, and that she would be less likely to ask for what she wants out of worries that he would think she was strange. But others tell me that sometimes one of the two really wants it to turn into a relationship and ends up getting hurt. A friend with benefits may become jealous if the other person gets involved with someone else, but may feel like they can't talk about it because getting attached isn't supposed to be part of the deal.

You might want to talk about these issues with your friend before embarking on something that might be more complicated than it appears.

I am in special classes at school because of a learning disability. For some of my courses, including gym, I am with what they call the "general population." Part of gym is health class. Right now we are doing sex education. I think our teacher is pretty embarrassed by the material, and he often has us read stuff instead of talking about it. I am too embarrassed to raise my hand and explain that I don't understand the stuff we are supposed to read, but I would really like to know some of it. He keeps on talking about how important it is to use condoms, but we had to read about how to use one.

You are right that this is information you should have. I can think of a few possibilities for how to learn more about sex, but for most of them you will have to ask, which you have said is hard for you. Keep telling yourself how important it is to get the information.

Start with the Internet. Sex, Etc. (www.sexetc.org) has a lot of good videos, although they aren't specific to disability or chronic health conditions. I wouldn't recommend doing a more general Internet search, but you can trust links from this site.

Once you have learned what you can from these resources (or if you don't have access to the Internet that gives you some privacy), a school nurse may be able to help with this. You can ask him in private, which is a bit easier than in front of a class. Some schools have school-based clinics, and one of their main jobs is to give information about protecting yourself from sexually transmitted infections (STI).

Your local public health department probably runs family planning and STI clinics. Often, you don't even need an appointment. You can call the department to find out where the clinics are. They are happy to provide information.

There may be a clinic in your town or city which is just for teens. You can find out about it by asking the school nurse or a guidance counselor.

Sometimes people have a class where, whatever the subject is supposed to be, they can ask questions about anything. If you have a teacher who likes to have discussions about many things, you may be able to bring up some of this. You may be able to say "Mr. So and So says we should know how to use condoms, but he doesn't tell us how." There is a good chance that the other people in your special classes also haven't understood the information they are getting in health class.

If someone is reading this book to you, he or she might be able to give you some information, or help you find the resources you need.

Parents vary in their willingness to talk about sex. If you think one of your parents would feel OK about giving you this information, and you feel comfortable hearing it from them, then this would be a good way to find out what you want to know.

> **I'm a 17-year-old guy with spina bifida. I have fallen in love with another guy. At first, I thought it was the worst thing in the world that could happen to me, but I feel so happy when I'm with him that I've realized it can't be such a bad thing. We've kissed and touched, but that's all. We both want to do more, but he's afraid he will hurt me or something, and I'm not sure what I'm capable of.**

I'm sure you're capable of a lot, and I wouldn't demean kissing and touching, both of which can be very important in a sexual relationship. Because of your spina bifida, sex might be more complicated for you than for some other teens, depending on how much function and feeling you have.

You may have some feeling in your penis, no feeling in your penis or full feeling in your penis. You may or may not have erections. The amount of anal sensation you have may vary. You probably know most of this information about yourself already, but a good place to start with your partner would be to map this out. Have him explore your sensation with his hands or tongue. You will have some areas that are more sensitive than others. You'll want to explore his body the same way.

If you are considering anal intercourse, it is important to remember that this is very high-risk behavior for transmitting HIV and other infectious agents. It is important that whoever is putting their penis into someone's anus use a condom and lube, as this will really decrease the risk. If you have decreased sensation in the area, be especially cautious, as these delicate tissues can be harmed by excessive pressure and friction. If you have erections, there is no barrier to anal intercourse with him as the receiving partner (as long as you wear a condom). Lots of gay men don't have anal intercourse—it isn't something you have to do to be able to call yourself gay.

There is much more to male sexuality than penises, and your body is covered with erogenous zones. Everyone is unique in their areas of maximum pleasure, but common ones are earlobes, nipples, lips and tongues. Even if you have no erections and no feeling in your penis, you can still have pleasurable, exciting sexual relations utilizing these areas. Remember that your brain is the most powerful sexual organ you have. Thinking and talking about sex are important parts of sexuality.

After my accident I was in the hospital for a long time because I had a head injury and had to learn how to do a lot of stuff again. My girlfriend visited me a lot once I was in rehab. I really wanted to have sex but she said we had to wait until I was out of the hospital. When I got home I told her it was time for us to have sex and she said that she didn't feel ready yet. I yelled at her and I was really mad because she had pretty much promised that we would have sex when I wasn't in the hospital anymore. Now she says she definitely won't have

sex with me if I yell at her like that again. I feel like I really need to get some sex and don't know how I'm going to get it.

Having a head injury can have an effect on your relationships and your sex life.

Many teens change after a head injury. Your girlfriend may feel that she is in a relationship with a different person from before and wants to get to know you better before getting back to your sexual relationship. It might be helpful to ask her if she is feeling this way and to ask her what the two of you can do to get connected again. You may be finding it harder to communicate these days, so planning out what to say, maybe even writing it down, could be helpful. Talk to one of your therapists about how to control your impulse to yell at or do other scary things to your girlfriend.

Some teens find that after a head injury they want to have sex a lot more than they did before; some have the opposite feelings. It sounds like you are feeling very strong sexual desires. This is fine, but you don't have a right to get lots of sex with other people just because you want it. Your feelings of needing sex may be so powerful that you aren't considering your girlfriend's feelings. She may feel you are trying to push her into something that she doesn't want to do. I assume that you are masturbating regularly. Remember that it is important to find a private place for this.

It may be that you have changed so much that you and your girlfriend aren't really right for each other anymore. She may even be feeling this already. It might be time for you to suggest taking a break from the relationship, and you can start looking for someone new.

I keep getting into these bad situations and I don't know how to stop it from happening. I was in a car accident two years ago and had what they call a TBI (traumatic brain injury). I'm back in school, and I just want to have the same kind of life my friends do. We go to the mall after school and guys come over and talk to us. They give us their phone numbers and my friends tell them that they will call. But when I have called one of these guys, he has thought that I would have sex with him. This has happened a few times now, and not just with the same guy. And a couple of them have made me do stuff that I didn't like. I thought maybe one would be my boyfriend, but none ever called again. I don't want to ask my friends how to stop this from happening because I don't think it happens to them. What can I do?

Sometimes after a brain injury it can be harder to figure out what is safe and to plan ahead for situations. It sounds like this is happening to you.

It may be that your friends never actually call these guys because they know it isn't always safe. It is hard for anyone to judge who is safe and who isn't just by chatting with them for a while at the mall. Some guys assume that if a girl they don't know calls them up and wants to get together, this is because she wants to have sex.

If you meet a guy who you want to get to know better, you could see if a friend of yours liked one of his friends and see about getting together in a group. Tell your friend that you don't want to have sex and make a pact that you won't leave each other alone with one or both guys.

It is also safer to get to know guys who go to your school. You will have seen how they act toward girls and talk about them. Your friends might have heard what they are like. This does not totally protect you, but it is a start.

Never go with a guy to any isolated place or his home unless you have been going out (in person) for quite a while and are sure you can trust him.

The last time I went to my doctor, she saw that my hair was dyed and said I should make sure that the hairdresser uses plastic, not latex, gloves, because I might be allergic to the latex. She said that this was because I did intermittent catheterization for several years. Why is this, and does it mean I can't use condoms?

Latex is a substance produced from the sap of rubber trees. For some reason, one group of people who seem to be at high risk for latex allergy is people with spina bifida who have used intermittent catheterization. As rubber is a plant product, it is not surprising that people can develop allergies to it. The reaction is thought to be from impurities in the rubber rather than from the latex polymer itself. The theory is that your mucous membranes (which are not as tough as the rest of your skin) have been exposed to latex on many occasions, and that this could lead to an allergy developing. In addition, if you have had surgery, the cut surfaces have been exposed to latex.

People with latex allergies can have severe reactions to latex products, including condoms. Hives—an itchy, splotchy, red rash—are probably the most common reaction, but people can also get wheezing and even a serious allergic reaction called anaphylaxis, which can kill you.

Not everyone who has had lots of mucous membrane contact with latex has a latex allergy. You can get tested for this, but while you are waiting for the testing you should consider not using latex condoms or a diaphragm. If you are having a pelvic or rectal exam, ask the doctor to use plastic gloves. Don't blow up balloons. Ask your dentist not to use latex dental dams (these are thin sheets of latex that may be used during dental work). If you have noticed a rash or itching after exposure, be especially careful about this. If you are in a situation where you are going to have intercourse and the only method of contraception available is condoms, much of the protein to which you might be allergic can probably be gently washed off a non-lubricated condom. After your partner has put the condom on his erect penis, wash it with a wet, warm washcloth (not your bare hand). This may be an enjoyable sensation for him, so consider it part of foreplay. After washing you can apply a water-soluble lubricant. For males with an allergy, the inside should be washed. Do this only in an emergency, as washing of latex has been tested only on gloves. There is also a risk of making a small hole—a potentially big problem!

If you avoid latex condoms and diaphragms and use other forms of birth control, you still have to worry about sexually transmitted infections (STIs). There are condoms made from polyurethane and others made from polyisoprene. They don't cause allergic reactions and protect against STIs and pregnancy. They are more expensive than latex condoms. Some people complain that the polyurethane ones make a crinkly noise when they have sex. The only brands of polyisoprene condoms available in North America are Skyn or Durex Avanti brands. Trojan Supra are polyurethane condoms.

The female condom is inserted into the vagina and held in place by rings inside and outside the vagina. In the US and Canada, the female condom that is currently available is made of synthetic nitrile. Nitrile isn't thought to cause allergic reactions, but there have been concerns about latex contamination of nitrile gloves and of reactions to some additives in them. You should be safe with nitrile female condoms. They are all made by one company, with different brand names in different places. The names you are likely to see are Reality and FC2. Polyurethane female condoms seem to have been phased out, which is too bad, as they were totally safe. A latex female condom is available in other countries and might come to North America soon, so don't assume that all female condoms are safe for you.

Another option is to avoid penetrative sex—that is, vaginal or anal intercourse. Although some people have the idea that only intercourse is real sex, this isn't the case and with non-penetrative sex you can avoid many of the hazards of intercourse.

It seems that everything I hear about sex from my teachers, my doctor and my parents involves the word "don't." "Don't have sex," "Don't get pregnant," "Don't let anyone exploit you," "Don't have sex without a condom" and on and on. Aren't there some "dos"?

We adults often wonder why teens and young adults aren't sexually healthier. It isn't surprising when all we give them are negative messages about sex.

You will discover your own list of "dos" as you learn about yourself as a sexual being. Here are some ideas to get you thinking:

1. Get to know your body. Find out where your sensitive areas are. Learn to feel good about having sexual feelings. When

you masturbate, you are figuring out what feels good, and you are doing something that is just for you.

2. Learn to love your body. It gives you life, and even if it gives you pain, it can also bring you pleasure. You do not have to look like a model to have appreciation for your body.

3. Allow yourself to have sexual fantasies. Just because you fantasize about something does not mean you are going to try it.

4. Expect respect from potential sexual partners. Give them the respect they deserve.

5. Participate only in those sexual acts that you feel comfortable doing. Give yourself permission to enjoy what you choose to do.

6. Always have safer sex. This means protecting yourself by knowing what you want and don't want, using birth control if your lovemaking includes heterosexual intercourse and using a condom to prevent the spread of sexually transmitted diseases.

7. Tell your partner what you want. He or she can't be expected to read your mind.

8. Understand that when your partner says no, he or she means it.

I am a girl with congenital adrenal hyperplasia. I have been feeling really attracted to my best friend. Does this mean I'm a lesbian? If so, is it because I have CAH?

You might be a lesbian, but it certainly isn't for sure. Many people who eventually identify as gay or lesbian may be attracted to someone of the opposite sex sometimes, and people who are straight may find someone of the same sex attractive. The way to know if you are a lesbian is by paying attention to your sexual fantasies and who you are attracted to generally. Over time, these will give you a fairly clear message. That message might be that you are bisexual, lesbian or heterosexual.

More women with CAH are lesbians than women who don't have it. This is probably related to higher levels of testosterone, which is a hormone that both men and women have but that is usually much higher in men than women. In general, there doesn't seem to be a scientific "cause" for homosexuality, although research suggests that those with a family member that is gay are more likely to be gay themselves.

When a young person is attracted to someone of the same sex, they can feel anxious, confused, happy, excited … many feelings are possible. Some of how you feel will be because of what you have heard about lesbians or gay men as you were growing up. If your parents have said negative things, then you are more likely to be worried about the possibility of being gay. Sometimes young people get so worried about this that they think about killing themselves. If you are scared or worried or confused, you should find someone you can talk with about this.

I have kidney disease and I rarely have a period— maybe two or three times a year. I will be going on dialysis soon. Will this make my periods come back?

Most young women with chronic renal failure have few or no periods due to a complex interaction of their illness and the parts of the brain that control the menstrual cycle.

It is hard to predict the effect of going on dialysis. Some young women tell me that they started having regular periods after a few months on dialysis, and this may happen to you. Others have few periods while on dialysis.

If your periods become regular on dialysis, you might be ovulating, which means that you could get pregnant if you have sex. Keep this in mind. Even if you have only the occasional period, you never know when you are going to ovulate, so don't assume that you are not fertile. If you think you might be pregnant, the reliable way to diagnosis it is with an ultrasound. A pregnancy test may be positive in a woman who is on dialysis when she isn't actually pregnant. This can cause a lot of anxiety for no reason.

I have bad arthritis in my hands. In a joke gift exchange, someone gave me a vibrator. I was secretly thrilled, but it hasn't worked out that well. It is hard to hold and those pesky little switches don't help. Also, the vibrations can make my joints hurt. Does anyone make sex toys for people like me?

Some people are interested in sex toys, some aren't. Sex toys can be homemade (like a feather duster to tickle your skin, or using a stream of water to stimulate yourself) and can be used when alone or with a partner.

Most sex-toy makers don't emphasize accessibility or ease of use in their product lines. There are a few who purposely do, and others who accidentally make a really user-friendly sex toy.

There are several choices to make when buying a vibrator (probably the most popular sex toy). Some are penis shaped and meant for insertion into either the vagina or the rectum. Others are meant for stimulation of the clitoris or nipples and come in a variety of shapes (including a rubber ducky—easy to conceal!). Many women don't find a vaginal vibrator all that interesting, but the penis-shaped ones can be used on other parts of your body. Vibrators can be made of metal, plastic, latex rubber or silicone. A silicone vibrator will last a long time, can be boiled (if it is a sealed unit) and is more expensive than the other types. Plastic vibrators (usually the cheapest types) may have seams that can scratch.

As you have discovered, there can be switches on vibrators that are difficult to manipulate. There are a number with remote controls, either connected with a wire (less expensive) or not (more pricey). You would have to look at these to see which have controls you could use easily. At the time of writing, there is only one, very expensive, Bluetooth-enabled vibrator (called "The Toy"), shaped like a large capsule. Designed for insertion, you could hold it against your vulva by squeezing your thighs around it. It is out of the typical adolescent price range. There are vibrators with switches that you press on and off, rather that switching back and forth. Quite a few vibrators are designed for hands-free use.

Other sex toys include dildos (penis shaped, no vibration) for penetration, insertion toys (for guys) and, as I mentioned, endless possibilities of objects around the house. Make sure you never use anything with rough or sharp edges, and don't put anything inside you that doesn't have a string or other way of getting it out, and make sure it is clean first.

Access to sex toys can be a problem for young people. Many places have laws that limit the sale of sex toys to people over the age of 16, 18 or even 21. Some vibrators are marketed as massagers and are available at department stores or places that sell various electrical gadgets. There are some excellent online sex-toy stores, with reviews and information on their websites (see the Resources section), but you might not want your dad opening up the mysterious package that comes addressed to you! If at all possible, order from a store that ships from your country so as not to get your package stopped at the border.

One of the guys I met at the HIV clinic says that he doesn't think you have to tell anyone you have sex with that you are HIV-positive. He says it is that person's responsibility to insist that you use a condom, and that if they don't, whatever happens is their fault. I haven't had sex with anyone and I don't plan to anytime soon, but I wonder what you think of this.

You can probably imagine what I think of this. Yes, everyone should insist that condoms be used before having penetrative sex. However, if they do not, because they don't know enough to, are scared to bring it up or even if they just don't care, they should not be given a sexually transmitted infection as a consequence. I think you have a responsibility to protect your partner, and I think what this guy is doing is wrong.

Are you required to tell? In many places it is illegal to have penetrative sex with someone without having told them your HIV positive status. It can be considered to be an assault, and people have gone to jail for this. Even if this isn't the case where you live, we know that condoms aren't foolproof. My feeling is that if you are doing anything that can lead to giving someone the virus (like vaginal or anal intercourse, even with a condom), your partner should be told. If you are doing safer things (like hugging and kissing), then I don't think you have to tell. But if you don't trust the person enough to confide about something that has had a big impact on your life, do you trust the person enough to be doing anything else with him or her?

It is probably a bad idea to tell someone this out of the blue. Find ways to make sure the person has realistic information about HIV. Ask hypothetical questions (e.g., "Would you go out with someone who is HIV-positive?") to see how the person feels. When you decide to talk about it, be in a place where you feel comfortable talking, and where you won't have to worry about being overheard.

As you tell people about your condition, you will get a variety of reactions. Some people will be supportive and, unfortunately, some will be freaked out. Life may get both harder and easier for you as more people know. People may talk about you, and some ignorant types will avoid you or say nasty things. On the other hand, you will not have the burden of keeping it secret and you will know who your real friends are.

I'm a girl but I don't have a vagina, I have a condition known as MRKH. My mother says it is really important that I get a vagina. I went to the gynecologist who explained that because I have a little bit of a vagina, I probably won't need surgery. She told me that I would have to use dilators regularly to make a vagina and keep it "working." It seems like a lot of hassle to me. I don't have a burning desire to have intercourse at this time. Is there a medical reason why I shouldn't wait until I feel more ready for the surgery?

MRKH is one of the few conditions left that has people's names attached to it. It stands for Mayer-Rokitansky-Küster-Hauser syndrome. People with MRKH don't have a uterus (see the section on pregnancy for more on this) and either have no vagina or just a bit of one. A vagina can be made with dilators or with surgery plus dilators. Dilators are like smooth plastic candles and come in different sizes. You would begin with the small size, about the size of a pen, and then move on to larger sizes. You press the dilator into the little bit of vagina that you have with a steady pressure (not so hard that it hurts). Some people say having a warm bath first relaxes the area but this adds to the time the process takes—and it does require a fairly big time commitment. Most doctors say you should use the dilators for 20 minutes twice a day, and that it can take up to six months of regular use for results. The time is worth it if you really want more of a vagina, but not if you don't.

There is no critical time period to make a vagina, and it is safe to wait until you think you will need a vagina or want to have one. If you agree to do it to make your mother happy, it is likely that you won't remember to do it regularly or will skip it frequently when there are more important things to do. Then your mother will nag you, and you'll fight with her. It won't be pretty.

It sounds like your mother has a hard time accepting that you don't have a vagina. She may think that you don't see yourself as feminine without one. It may seem like an essential piece of equipment for any woman to have.

Tell your mother that you want to go back to see the gynecologist with her. Talk to the doctor alone first and ask her to meet with your mother to discuss her feelings about this and to explain to her that a vagina isn't needed to make you a girl. She can help your mother understand that it is OK to wait until you are ready.

I have a colostomy and I can't imagine having sex with anyone. I mean, the bag could fall off or fill up, and it would just be too embarrassing. So I've just decided that I'm not going to get it on with anyone. Maybe when I'm old I won't care about that kind of stuff, so then I could have sex—when I'm in my 30s or something.

Although I'm not saying you should rush out and get into a sexual relationship today, I do think you are limiting your life possibilities by taking such a firm stand on this.

Most people with ostomies worry about smells, sounds, appearance and the bag coming off during sex. But, many people with ostomies have learned ways to minimize these risks and enjoy having sex as part of their lives.

Although it may be hard to tell a potential partner about your ostomy, it is probably a good idea to do so before he or she discovers it. If you present it as not a big deal, your partner is more likely to accept it. Unless your surgery was recent and you are still healing, you do not have to worry about the pressure on your ostomy from a partner lying on you or pressing against you.

If your bag doesn't usually leak, you probably have a well-fitting appliance that is sticking well. You may want to put some tape around the edges for extra security. You can empty the pouch before you think you are going to have sex, which will reduce the risk of leaking and increase your level of comfort (as you won't have to worry about it sloshing about).

Avoid positions that put pressure on the bag or move the bag, as they increase the risk of it coming off. Putting a sash or scarf around your waist will lessen the chance of the bag falling off, will cover it up and will decrease noise. Don't get too uptight about noises—your non-ostomate partner may also fart while you are having sex, or just after.

If you think you might be having sex, don't eat foods the same day that produce a lot of gas or that seem to go through you quickly. I suspect you've figured out which foods do this to you.

Your stoma should never be penetrated with anything as part of sex.

If your rectum was removed as part of your surgery, this may affect your sexual response. Muscles around your rectum that contract during orgasm may have been removed or weakened. If you have leakage from your anus, you will want to clean the area before sex (maybe shower with your partner). If you are a girl, your vagina and uterus may move into a different position, causing different sensations. If scar tissue near the vagina causes pain during intercourse, extra lubrication with a water-based lubricant may help. You may wish to try different positions or sexual practices that don't involve penetration.

If you are a guy and are having trouble getting an erection after surgery, you need to consider both physical and psychological factors. If you have an ileostomy, you are unlikely to have erectile difficulty as a result. On the other hand, urostomies often result in not being able to have erections. Many men who have a physical cause for soft or absent erections can still have orgasms. If you sometimes have an erection when you wake up in the morning, then problems having erections during sex are more likely to be from anxiety, worries about your stoma and appliance, depression, medication or alcohol. Remember that many potential partners are happy to have non-penetrative sex.

How do you actually talk with someone about sex? I have a hard time even writing this and I know that if I had to use any sex words, my face would turn red, my mouth would get dry and I wouldn't know what to say. You say that talking about sex is important and my phys ed teacher says in health class that you have to "negotiate" condom use, but I don't know where to start.

The first thing is to make sure that you know what words to use and what they mean. You can get this information from a trustworthy website, like Go Ask Alice!, About.com or Sex, Etc. (see the Resources section for the URLs).

Then you can start practicing by yourself. Find a private spot and say all those sex words that you are worried about.

Say them by themselves first, then make up sentences using them. Then do the same thing while you are looking in a mirror. When this becomes easier, you can move on to the next stage. Sometimes it is easier to bring up a topic that you find difficult when you don't have to make eye contact. If you are alone in a car with the person you want to talk with, this is a great opportunity, as one of you will be keeping their eyes on the road. A dim room is another option, or while out for a walk. Starting a sentence with, "I've been wondering..." or something like that is good. If you know what you want to talk about, write some of it down first and read it over, first silently to yourself and then out loud. You can't take this script with you to the conversation, though, unless this is the usual way you communicate with this person. Have an idea of what it is you want to accomplish with the conversation. Do you want to get information, convey information, tell someone how you feel or let them know what you want? Knowing this will help you stay on track.

Even if things don't go exactly as planned, see this as more practice rather than as a disaster.

I have pulmonary hypertension (PH). I have been dating someone for a while and we are moving toward a more sexual relationship. But it seems complicated. I'm on oxygen; can I take it off as long as I am lying down? And what about my line for getting IV prostacyclin? I'm worried it will fall out or something.

I can promise you that you won't be the first person with PH to have sex. Thinking about this in advance is a good idea.

If you need oxygen, you need it while you are having sex. Nasal prongs shouldn't interfere with kissing or oral sex. If you or your partner get a bit tangled up in the tubing, try to see it as more funny than embarrassing.

Although you are unlikely to pull out your line having sex, you should not lie directly on it or let it get squished between the two of you.

Depending on how severe your condition is, you might find that you run out of energy pretty quickly. Taking a nap before sex might be a good idea. Young people with PH have told me that things work well when they take their time—lots of cuddling, kissing, and so on. You might want to look into tantric yoga, which involves minimal exertion and, I have heard, great orgasms.

You may find that lying flat on your back with someone on top of you makes you feel short of breath. Also, if you are on top there is less chance of your tubing getting kinked. Other positions to consider are lying on your side or having sex in a chair or on the sofa.

If you take pain medication, take some about half an hour before having sex (if you are planning that far in advance) or right before.

Like everyone else, if you can walk up two flights of stairs, you are unlikely to be restricted in how active you are when you have sex. If you can't, you will probably automatically adjust to a level of activity that works for you.

OK, what's the bottom line? Can I have sex or not?

Everyone can have sex. Not everyone can have sexual intercourse, and intercourse may not be enjoyable for some people who can accomplish it. But (I repeat) everyone can have sex. Sex that does not include intercourse is still real sex.

You probably wouldn't be asking this question if we lived in a society where people with illnesses or disabilities weren't seen as being asexual. What lies behind this attitude isn't clear to me. What is the benefit to our culture as a whole to have a group of people who are regarded as being unable to have sex? Maybe it's that people with chronic conditions are viewed as being perpetual children, and we tend to view children as asexual (another myth). Whatever it is, it is an idea that is widespread, unspoken, untrue and destructive to how people feel about themselves.

Even many parents think this way. They will tell doctors that their child doesn't need to know anything about sex or birth control, because they are sure their child will never have sex. (Some parents of kids without a disability or illness also can't think of their children as being potentially sexual, but this isn't as common.)

All of us are created as sexual beings. There are great differences in levels of sexual desire and in levels of sexual activity. There are special considerations with some conditions, but they don't mean you can't have sex.

A definition of sex that is broader than just intercourse is something we as a culture need to adopt. Surveys have shown that many women get more pleasure from sexual activities other than intercourse. Intercourse is also a high-risk behavior in the transmission of sexually transmitted infections. Intercourse can lead to pregnancy. A focus on sex as intercourse is (in my opinion) the basis for high numbers of unwanted pregnancies, sexually transmitted infections and people who are unhappy with their sex lives.

Having sex with yourself is not a "second best" option. It is a good way to get to know your capabilities and does not carry the risk that intercourse does. If you have difficulty using your hands or controlling your movements, you may be able to masturbate by using a vibrator (available by catalog and in many stores) or by positioning yourself so a spray of water from a shower or hose in the bathtub hits your genitals. Water should not be sprayed into the vagina. Some people find that it enriches their sexual fantasies to read erotica (sexy books), watch films with sex scenes or look at pictures. Only do what you feel comfortable doing. Explore as much of your body as you can. There can be sexual feeling in many places, including ears, the neck and nipples (for guys too!).

Here are some special considerations for specific conditions (listed alphabetically). Drugs that can cause changes in sexual interest or sexual functioning are listed in Appendix 1. Birth control considerations are discussed later in the chapter.

Amputation: If this occurred before you were a teen, it is unlikely to cause any problems. Your methods for adapting to a missing limb in other parts of your life will probably flow naturally into adaptations for sexuality.

If your amputation is more recent, dealing with your feelings about the amputation is important, as depression and other emotional problems can lead to sexual problems. If you have had an arm or hand amputated that you previously used to masturbate or to stimulate a partner, you may need to practice for a while before being as comfortable or skilled with your other hand. If your stump is still healing or has a sensitive area on it, you will want to find positions that avoid pressure on the area. This may mean being on the bottom or lying on your side. Most people find that a prosthesis gets in the way, so they take it off before or during lovemaking.

You should know that there are people whose sexual attractions are toward people with amputations. You may come in contact with such a person. People have different feelings about this. One teen told me that she thinks it's great: "If a guy was attracted to me because I have blonde hair or because I play the cello, I wouldn't mind that. Why would I mind it that he finds my amputation attractive?" Others have said that they want someone to be attracted to them for who they are, not their physical attributes.

Anemia: If you are very anemic, or have had anemia for a long time, you may have less sexual drive as part of your fatigue. If you get regular blood transfusions, take advantage of your increased energy in the week after the transfusion. If you have an illness that results in a treatable anemia, your sex drive should come back as you become less anemic.

Arthritis—Juvenile Idiopathic Arthritis (JIA): If your JIA is well controlled, you may experience no difficulties. Depending on which joints are affected, the impact on your sex life will vary.

You may find that you get pain in your jaw (in the joint up near your ear) when you kiss or have oral sex. Kiss for short periods of time with other activities in between.

You may find that your hands are too stiff to use them as you would like. Try using the back of your hand to stroke your lover. You can also caress him or her with your face, your chest and your hair. When masturbating, you may want to use aids such as a vibrator or a stream of water.

If dry eyes and mouth are part of their illness, females may notice that their vagina is dry too. This can lead to pain during intercourse. Use a water-based lubricant (you or your partner can put it on your vulva or on his penis or his or her fingers).

During intercourse, you may find that pressure on affected joints will hurt. Find positions that avoid this (like lying on your side either facing toward each other or "spooned") and prop up the joint with a pillow so that it is supported.

If you have limited motion in a joint, you may need to find a position that will accommodate this. Both men and women can have intercourse with knees and/or hips that will not bend or straighten. Females may want to try having their legs hanging over the end of the bed with their partner kneeling on the floor.

Fatigue and pain can decrease sex drive and make sex something of a challenge. Having sex increases the amount of cortisol (like prednisone) that your body makes, so sex may help alleviate arthritis pain. Position yourself carefully and prop up affected joints with pillows to prevent pain. Having a hot bath before sex may help you relax the muscles around your joints. Arthritis in the hands can make it difficult to put on a condom or hold a sex toy. The female condom might be easier to use.

Asthma: You probably won't experience any difficulties having sex that relate to your asthma. If you have exercise-induced asthma and find that you wheeze during or after sex, you can use your puffer to prevent this. Use your puffer when preparing for sex, for instance, when the other person is putting on a condom or putting one on you.

Blindness/Visual Impairment: Your sexual functioning should not be affected by your condition. Although erotic films and pictures aren't accessible (and the sound tracks for films are pretty bad), there are other options. There is so much free erotica on the Internet (and even more available as e-books) that as long as you have screen-reading software, an e-reader, and a pair of headphones, you have access to a great deal of fantasy material. And a partner who can see may get into reading erotic stories to you.

Cancer: Some brain tumors may influence your level of sexual desire. If there is an increase, your partner may not want to have sex more often than you do already. You may need to increase the amount you masturbate. If your sexual desire is reduced, it will be helpful for your partner to know that this isn't because you find him or her less attractive. There may be times when you are willing to have sex to please your partner even when you don't desire it. This is fine, but if it becomes the pattern of your sexual relationship, you may start to feel resentful.

Chemotherapy may make you feel less attractive, especially if you lose your hair. Your partner may find you just as attractive with less hair, so don't make assumptions. Wigs can fall off during sex. If you are going to worry about this, it will interfere with your pleasure, so consider removing it beforehand. If chemotherapy makes you feel nauseated, you are unlikely to want to have sex until you are feeling better. Explain this to your partner.

Pelvic radiation treatments can cause damage to the vaginal wall, leading to discomfort or pain during intercourse. It can also lead to problems with erection and painful ejaculation. If you can get your radiation oncologist alone in a private spot, you can ask about this.

Cerebral Palsy with Athetosis: Sometimes, difficulties in controlling your movements may make masturbation and caressing your partner challenging, although these movements in the tongue can be quite stimulating during kissing and oral sex. You need a partner who can have a sense of humor about getting bopped occasionally. Your partner can caress you and stimulate you in a number of ways. If your movements make it impossible to get physically close enough to have sex, you can still be with your partner while you both masturbate (perhaps using the sex toys mentioned above), watch movies or talk about sex.

Cerebral Palsy with Spasticity: You may find that your spasms vary, depending on how relaxed and comfortable you are with your partner. If they are fairly mild, you may just need to take your time and find positions that help you relax. A warm bath before (or as part of) sex may reduce spasms.

If you take medication to reduce spasms, consider asking your doctor if you can take extra before having sex.

Trying different positions for intercourse can be useful. Women with spasticity in their hip adductors (which makes the legs stay together) find that vaginal penetration is easier from behind. If you are a guy who can't straighten his legs, try having intercourse with your partner on top, leaning back against your bent legs. If they are bent right up to your belly, sometimes partial penetration can happen with your partner on top of your legs.

If you have a lot of spasticity, intercourse may be difficult or even impossible. Even if your legs are relaxed, muscle spasms can occur in the vaginal muscles, interfering with penetration and causing pain. Stimulating each other with your hands or mouths may be more workable, and you can also masturbate with each other, watch sexy movies or talk about sex.

Congenital Adrenal Hyperplasia: Males with CAH may have a penis that is larger than average, although this doesn't usually present any problems. Females may have an enlarged clitoris. This does not interfere with sexual function, but it may be something you want to mention to someone before they discover it for themselves. Some women also have a smaller than average vaginal opening, which can make intercourse challenging. This can often be adjusted with the use of vaginal dilators or surgery, if it is important to you.

Cystic Fibrosis: You may find that having sex leads to increased coughing. Have something on hand (a plastic bag or a mug) to help deal with all the mucus. Partners who are warned about this are more likely to deal with this well. If you find that coughing relates to certain positions or activity levels during sex, you can modify these. You may find it difficult to breathe with someone lying on top of you. If so, you can either adjust positions so you are never on the bottom or have the other person support their weight on their arms or elbows.

Decreased sexual desire is fairly common and can be dealt with by planning to have sex at times when you know you have more energy, and by trying to tune in to subtle cues that you are feeling sexual.

Girls and women may not have very much vaginal lubrication when they are excited. The secretions from your vagina are thicker than those of someone without CF. In addition, these secretions may be affected by your being on antibiotics frequently. There are numerous lubricants on the market. If you find that intercourse is painful or uncomfortable, consider using one. You can coat your lover's fingers or penis with lubricant as part of having sex, or have your partner put it on you.

Don't assume that you are less attractive because you may be shorter or thinner than your friends. People are attracted to a variety of features in potential partners. They are more likely to be attracted to someone who makes them feel wanted and more alive.

Deafness/Hearing Impairment: If your partner can hear, you may need to remind them that you can't hear what they whisper in your ear. However, much communication while making love is non-verbal.

Diabetes: Some boys and men may have difficulty getting erections. Although this can have a physical cause (peripheral neuropathy), it is more likely to be psychological and involve how they feel about themselves and their illness. Hypoglycemia can cause temporary problems with getting erections.

Vaginal yeast infections are more common in girls and women with diabetes. Mild infections may not have any effect, but more severe ones can lead to pain during or after intercourse or even after masturbation. Yeast infections should be treated before they get to that point. Prevent and treat yeast infections with lactobacillus acidophillus capsules. This is the bacteria used to make yogurt and is available at many health food stores. The capsules should be kept in a cool place (the refrigerator is best). Insert one capsule (they are small) into your vagina every night for a week after your period. If this doesn't work, try using them every night. The only possible complication is if you accidentally put one into your urethra (the opening you pee out of). This will hurt. Just go to the bathroom and pee. Even a few drops should make the capsule come out.

Some adult women with diabetes say that their orgasms become less intense with age and find that using a vibrator helps.

Heart Disease: If you have the energy to walk up two flights of stairs, then you probably will experience no problems with having sex. If you do have severely decreased energy, you can modify your sexual activity to conserve energy. Take things a bit more slowly. If someone is on the bottom, make sure it is you. Stop and take a rest if you get chest pain.

Kidney Disease: People in chronic renal failure and not yet on dialysis are likely to have a decreased interest in sex. Boys and men may have difficulty getting and keeping erections, and girls and women may have problems attaining orgasm. They may lose their period, or get their first one later than their friends. Dialysis or transplantation often helps improve all these situations.

A combination of your disease and the treatment may have made you quite short. It can be a struggle to get people to see you as a teen instead of as a child. In addition, when you are having sex you will need to experiment with positions to adjust to whatever difference in size there is between you and your lover.

Depression can lead to a loss of interest in sex. If you are on dialysis and still are less interested in sex than you used to be (or would like to be), consider that depression may be causing this. If you think it is, find someone whom you can trust to talk with and try to work through this.

Lupus (SLE): The main problem you are likely to run into is fatigue, resulting in a lower sex drive. Some strategies dealing with fatigue and sex drive are discussed elsewhere in this chapter.

MRKH/Vaginal Agenesis: The outside part of your genitals isn't affected, so you can have orgasms and participate in any sexual activity except vaginal intercourse. If you want to have vaginal intercourse, there are a number of ways to get a vagina, including the regular use of dilators and several kinds of surgery. You'll find a question earlier in this chapter about this—read it for more info.

Multiple Sclerosis (MS): As this condition shows itself in a wide variety of ways, the effects on sexuality can also be varied. Most people with MS have normal levels of sexual interest, although depression and fatigue can limit your sexual desire.

Boys and men with MS may have difficulty in getting erections or in keeping them. Some have erections but don't have orgasms. If you have problems with erections, sexual activity can still include touching and stroking your partner and using your mouth and tongue to stimulate him or her. Your partner can do all these things too. You may find it pleasurable to have your penis touched even if you don't get an erection.

For both men and women, sensitivity in parts of your body may be affected. Your genitals may need more stimulation, or it may hurt to have them touched the way you were used to. The best thing to do is to experiment until you find out which parts of your body you enjoy having touched.

Also, in either gender, the ability to use your hands may be affected. You will need to be inventive about using other parts of your body to caress your partner. Masturbation can also be more difficult, and you may want to experiment with a spray of water directed at your genitals, a vibrator or rubbing against a pillow or stuffed animal.

Girls and women who have leg spasms, especially ones that bring their legs together, can have difficulty with intercourse. Any tricks they have learned to reduce spasm can be used, as can the alternatives to intercourse discussed above. (Also see the suggestions in the section above on cerebral palsy.)

If you have concerns about bladder control and are not on medication to help, you may want to discuss this with your partner. Sex may be a bit less spontaneous, as you will probably want to be on a bed with some protection. It's a good idea to pee before you make love. Sex in the bath or shower also gets around the problem. Sex tends to get pretty wet anyway, so a little extra may not be all that noticeable.

Muscular Dystrophy (MD): Puberty may start late if you have MD. Sometimes hormonal levels can be altered. If you are experiencing irregular menstrual cycles or big fluctuations in sexual desire, your doctor may be able to help. Males with decreased or no sexual desire should also talk to their doctor about hormone supplements.

Contractures and muscle weakness can complicate the mechanics of sex, but experimenting with alternatives to intercourse (touching, stroking, oral stimulation) and with different positions can lead to increased sexual pleasure.

Ostomy: See the question about sex and a colostomy, above.

Scoliosis: If you have severe scoliosis, some positions may be uncomfortable or impossible. You'll need to experiment to find comfortable positions.

Sickle Cell Anemia: A major problem can be decreased interest in sex, which results from being tired and not feeling well.

If you have joint problems, you may have to experiment with positions to find ones that are comfortable. You may find that using your hands in the same motion over and over bothers your wrists.

Spina Bifida and Spinal Cord Injury: This is addressed also in another question later in this chapter.

There is a lot of variation from person to person in skin and genital sensitivity and the ability of muscles to contract, depending on the level of spinal cord damage. If you feel comfortable asking, your doctor should be able to predict some of this for you.

For teens of both sexes, experimenting on your own and with your partner will help you discover which parts of your body are the most sexually sensitive. These areas can be concentrated on when having sex and may include the lips, earlobes, nipples, armpits, the inner elbow and the neck.

It is important to give yourself time to recover after a spinal cord injury. In the first year, many people have decreased sexual interest and abilities.

You may need to alter your bowel and/or bladder routine so that you don't have to worry about being incontinent while having sex. Sexual stimulation can increase the chance of incontinence. Having a bowel movement before going on a date and catheterizing before sex will prevent anxiety and help you feel more comfortable. Leg bags and catheters can be left on during sex, including intercourse. A catheter can be taped to the base of an erect penis.

Getting into a position where it is possible and comfortable to have sex is important. Transferring from your wheelchair and getting into a good position may require the help of an attendant, which can be difficult to negotiate as a teen. Your parents may be your only attendants, which puts a crimp in things. It is quite possible for people of any gender to have sex in a wheelchair. Removable armrests are a big plus for this. The other person can sit on your lap facing you or away from you. If the person in the chair is being penetrated, then sliding forward in the chair with their partner kneeling in front of them can be a good position.

Autonomic dysreflexia (AD) is a life-threatening condition that can occur in people with spinal cord injury during sex. It is rare but is more likely in people with an injury at or above T-6. It is more often triggered by a bladder infection, bowel problem or when a woman is in labor than by sex. It is more likely to be triggered by use of a vibrator than by other kinds of sexual activity. The warning signs for AD are increased spasticity, flushing and sweating. This can progress to blurred vision, headache, nasal congestion and nausea. Your body hair may stand on end. Have your partner help you into a position where your head is elevated, and call for medical help. **This is an emergency.**

Females: Girls with spina bifida tend to physically mature earlier than other girls. One effect of this is that you may be thinking about sex at a younger age than your friends. Girls with spinal cord injuries tend to lose their periods after the accident, but they usually return on their own.

You may have to experiment to find a good position for intercourse if your legs are paralyzed, as noted above. If you have no sensation in your genitals, intercourse may not bring any pleasure other than the pleasure of pleasing your partner and the feeling of shared intimacy. While you may want to do this sometimes, intercourse should not be the only basis for a sexual relationship, or things will be too one-sided. However, some women experience orgasms from having their cervix stimulated by a penis, finger or sex toy. The cervix is the part of the uterus that sticks out into the top of the vagina, and it can only be touched by something inserted into the vagina. If you are of legal age, it is up to you to decide if you want to try intercourse, but I wouldn't suggest that you do this as your very first sexual activity.

Even if you don't experience orgasms in your genitals, many people have orgasms that come from other parts of the body and involve the same elements of increased heart rate and breathing, swelling of the clitoris, labia and nipples, muscles tensing and relaxing, and a feeling of peace and relaxation afterward.

Males: The ability to have erections and to ejaculate varies from person to person. A majority of boys and men with spinal cord injuries are able to have erections, but many don't ejaculate. You are more likely to have erections if you have involuntary muscle contractions in your legs.

There are many alternatives for males who do not have erections. It is possible to "stuff" a penis that is not erect into a partner's vagina. Your partner can be pleasured when you caress her with your hands and your mouth. You can have your sensitive areas stimulated. Talking about sex before or while trying some of these alternatives can be exciting.

Remember that an inability to be physically dominant during sex does not mean you are passive. Being involved emotionally and seeing yourself as an active member of a sexual relationship will ensure that sex is not something that is done to you but is something in which you participate.

Transplants: Some people with kidney transplants worry that their kidney may be damaged if someone lies on them or puts pressure on their belly. You will not damage your new kidney transplant in this way—you probably sleep on your front sometimes and your weight doesn't hurt it then.

A more important concern for anyone who has had a transplant of any kind is protection from sexually transmitted infections. Always use condoms. Your medications suppress your immune response, which means that if you get an STI, the infection could be very serious, even life-threatening. Your partner needs to know that having sex with someone else and not telling you about it could kill you.

No matter what your disability or condition, if you have questions about sex that your doctor can't answer, think about asking him to help you start a support group for teens. Invite someone a bit older who has your condition and who is sexually active. He or she is likely to have lots of practical advice. The Resources section in Appendix 2 also lists online and print resources about sex.

I'm 19 and heading off for college at the end of the summer. This has been a big deal but it looks like all the details are working out. Up until now, my parents have been my attendants, except for a couple of times when they went away for a week-end. Now I will have attendants who are strangers. What help can I expect from them if I am going to have sex with someone? Can I just say, "I'm going out tonight, I might need you to get me ready and into bed fast so that I can have sex with my date?" There is no way I would want a girl I was going out with to do this for me.

Negotiating with attendants is a tricky thing. Most people have attendants who are employees of an agency (so the organization is the boss, not you), although some people have an arrangement where they are the boss. The agency might have rules about sex (almost for sure it has a rule that attendants can't have sex with clients), but these rules are often vague on what help can be offered around sex. Some people have had a hard time getting attendants to do anything to help them have sex, others have found attendants who will prop a vibrator in a good position, turn it on and leave the room.

It can be hard to talk about these things, but the only way you will get what you need is to ask for it. If you have an opportunity to interview your attendants before they are hired, this is a good time to bring up questions about privacy and to let them know that you plan to be dating. Remember that whoever this person is, they have their own issues around sexuality and have a unique view of sexuality that is based on what their parents have told them, their own experiences (that might not have been positive), their religious background and other factors.

Once you start dating someone, you can let your attendants know that that person might be coming back with you to the room sometimes. Ask them what they think would work best in terms of getting into bed. Things will vary from time to time. Sometimes you might want to have sex in your chair and then get into bed.

The person you are dating might not know a lot about attendant services and may not know what you need help with. You might have to explain what attendant services involve. If you think you might need help with positioning from the attendant before they leave, your partner may need some time to adjust to this idea. It is best if your partner can meet the attendant before there is any requirement for sexual assistance.

Be clear with the attendant about what you will need. Be as specific as you can. If you think that the attendant is feeling uncomfortable, you can bring this up. Let them know that you understand that this can be challenging and that you are happy to talk about it. You could also give them permission to talk to a colleague if they feel they need support. Assure them that you will not tell other attendants what they have said without permission.

**I have complex heart disease. I have been fool-
ing around with my boyfriend, but we haven't had
intercourse. Although I don't feel too bad, I know
that I'm not likely to live a long time, and I'd like
to have a full sex life while I still have some energy. I asked my doctor about the Pill, and he said
I couldn't take it. He also said I could die if I got
pregnant. He seemed to think that ended the discussion. What are my other options?**

Contraception, or birth control, comes in various forms. As
I'm sure you know, every month, changes in levels of hormones
produced by your pituitary gland (at the base of your brain)
stimulate your ovaries to release an egg. This egg travels through
your fallopian tube. If it meets and is fertilized by a sperm, it
will (usually) travel to your uterus and set up housekeeping
there. Contraceptives interfere with this process at any point.

The oldest methods of birth control are those that keep
the sperm and the egg apart. The most basic and effective is to
not have intercourse. Both males and females can be sexually
satisfied without intercourse, and this is a safe method of
pregnancy prevention. It sounds like you've ruled this out, but
you might want to reconsider. In another method, the rhythm
method, you calculate when you are likely to be fertile and
avoid having intercourse on those days. (Doctors like to joke
that people who rely only on the rhythm method are referred
to as "parents.") You can make this method more effective by
measuring and plotting your basal body temperature (your
temperature in the morning before you get out of bed) and
by examining your cervical mucus. The temperature part can
be a problem if you get a fever from an infection. Women with
cystic fibrosis usually can't use the mucus test, but you probably

could. If you are interested, check at Catholic hospitals, which often offer classes in these methods.

Barrier methods are contraceptive methods that prevent the sperm and the egg from meeting by providing a physical barrier. Because none of them are perfect (or even close), they should be used with a spermicide, a chemical that kills sperm. The most common barrier contraceptives are condoms used by the man, and diaphragms and cervical caps used by the woman.

A **condom** is a rubber (latex) or synthetic tube that fits over the erect penis, preventing the sperm from entering the vagina. You may have heard them called "rubbers," although most people just call them "condoms" these days. I have a patient whose boyfriend calls them "raincoats." Be careful to leave a bit of room at the end for the sperm to go into, and be sure not to make a hole in the condom when opening the package. Condoms can be bought at any drugstore without a prescription and have the additional advantage of lowering the chances of getting a sexually transmitted infection. Lately, condom manufacturers have been trying to make condoms more fun by spirals and extra material to increase the pleasure from penetration with a condom and also by making them in a variety of colors. Some people try one condom, don't like it and think they've tried them all. But there are differences between brands, so keep trying new ones until you find one you like. Use the condom from the beginning of intercourse, and use a new one every time you have intercourse.

Diaphragms and cervical caps are rubber cups that sit over the cervix. They are inserted through the vagina. The diaphragm is bigger and is easier to insert than the cervical cap. Both are used with spermicidal jelly. If you forget to take it out eight to twelve hours later, it could become a focus of infection. Diaphragms come in different sizes and you have to be fitted for one by a doctor or someone at a family planning clinic. Diaphragms and cervical caps do not prevent sexually transmitted infections and don't tend to be popular with young people.

The **contraceptive sponge** is a combination barrier and spermicide. You wet the small white sponge and put it in your vagina. Most sperm get trapped in the sponge, and the ones that don't get killed by the spermicide. It is best used with condoms. There have been problems getting the sponge manufactured, so it isn't available everywhere.

The **IUD or IUCD** (intrauterine contraceptive device) is a small piece of plastic that is inserted into the uterus by a doctor or other trained professional and is then left there. There are two kinds of IUDs used these days, both of which seem to work by making the uterus an unpleasant place for a fertilized egg to take root. The first has copper in it, which makes it more effective than just plain plastic. The copper IUD can bring heavy periods and bad cramps. The copper IUD has a failure rate a bit higher than that of the Pill, so condoms should be used too. In fact, anyone with an IUD should use condoms, as the IUD does not provide protection from sexually transmitted infections (STIs).

The other kind of IUD has progesterone (one of the sex hormones) in it that releases slowly over time. The brand name for this is Mirena. It is the most effective birth control there is. In the first few months, periods and other bleeding can be unpredictable, but by six months most women stop having periods (they come back when the IUD is removed).

Insertion of an IUD can be painful, as the uterus contracts when it senses something has entered it. Less commonly, there can be heart rate and rhythm changes, fainting and even seizures. The heart problems are minor in someone healthy but could be serious in someone with heart disease. If you have to take antibiotics before you have dental work, you should also do this for an IUD insertion. One of the biggest advantages of the IUD is that it can be left in for a long time—five years for the Mirena and even longer for the copper one. So once it is in, you don't have to worry about getting pregnant (although you still must use condoms to prevent STIs).

The **birth control pill** is a very effective female contraceptive device because it works in a number of ways. It usually prevents ovulation, but it also makes the uterus less hospitable to a fertilized ovum. It also changes cervical mucus and makes it more difficult for sperm to get through. The Pill must be taken every day. Most birth control pills used these days have very low doses of two types of hormones, progestins and estrogen. Some have equal amounts in each pill, others have variable amounts in an attempt to mimic the menstrual cycle. As you have said, the Pill is not an option for you: it can lead to pulmonary hypertension, increases the risk of embolism and can cause water retention. No one who has ever had a problem with blood clots should take the Pill.

Working exactly the same as the Pill is the **contraceptive patch**. Once a week for three weeks you put a new patch on your skin (not on your breast) and the medication is slowly released. The fourth week you don't use a patch and you get your period. If the patch comes off you have to replace it. This is a great option if you don't want to have to remember something every day. Also if you might have problems absorbing the pill, or if you have had a liver transplant, this is a good form of birth control. Whatever I say in this chapter about the Pill also applies to the patch.

Another variation on the Pill is the **vaginal ring**. It delivers the same two hormones through a little plastic ring-shaped tube that you put into your vagina once every three weeks. There is even less to remember than with the patch and it is a good method for those who don't feel uncomfortable inserting something into their vagina.

The **mini-pill** is a birth control pill that does not contain estrogen. Because of this, it is safer for people with vascular problems. It is not as effective in preventing pregnancy as the Pill and can cause irregular bleeding. It is important to take it at the same time every day.

Depo-Provera is a contraceptive that contains progesterone and is delivered in an injection. You get the shot once every three months. It is very effective in preventing pregnancy and is safer than the birth control pill (which is pretty safe itself). The advantage is that you only have to get the shot four times a year. In the first year on this method, your periods can be unpredictable. Some people bleed often, others don't. After the first year most girls and women don't get their period at all. It can take up to six months (some people say even longer) for fertility to return once the injections stop. However, a big concern is that it has been shown to decrease bone density. If this happens in healthy women, it seems likely that it could cause more problems in women with conditions or medications that already make bones weaker, and I tend not to recommend it to teens with these conditions or medications because of this.

Emergency contraception is something that is used if you have unprotected intercourse or if a condom breaks. It used to be called the "morning after pill," but there were people who thought they couldn't take it in the afternoon! There are two types, one that has estrogen and progesterone and the other with only progesterone (this one is called "Plan B"). This type with only one hormone is more effective and less likely to make you feel nauseated, and in many places it is available from a drugstore without a prescription. Some doctors will give their patients a prescription in advance to use if they need it. The two-hormone pills have to be taken twice, twelve hours apart. With Plan B two pills are taken at the same time.

If you feel you will never want to risk a pregnancy, you may want to choose **permanent sterilization**. Your fallopian tubes can be "tied" using a laparoscope. This instrument is inserted through very small incisions (cuts) in your abdomen with a local anesthetic, so it will be a low-risk procedure for you. It cannot be easily reversed, so you should think very carefully about it. If you decide to have this operation done, you may have a hard time finding a gynecologist who is willing to do it for someone of your age. However, if you have pulmonary hypertension (high blood pressure in your pulmonary artery), the operation can be quite tricky and should be performed only at a hospital where the anesthetists have experience with heart surgery.

For you, the safest bet is probably a barrier method with a spermicide. If you use a version of the rhythm method as well, you can increase your protection by avoiding intercourse when you are ovulating. If you think you are unlikely to use these methods every time you have intercourse, it might be wiser to use a more effective method, even if it is riskier for your health.

For people with other conditions, here is some contraceptive advice:

Allergies: Some women who take the birth control pill have reported increased sneezing, but I'm not aware of more serious allergic symptoms. It is therefore probably safe to start on the Pill and see if symptoms develop.

Another question in this chapter deals with latex allergies. If you have any reason to suspect a latex allergy, do not use latex condoms.

A number of people react to vaginal spermicides with itching and burning. This is probably not an allergic reaction.

A reaction to one spermicide preparation does not mean you will have a reaction to them all, so experiment a bit to find the right one for you.

Arthritis: The birth control pill is safe to use if you have arthritis. The pills are quite small, so if you have a lot of difficulty using your fingers you may have trouble with the pills. The containers they come in either have to be twisted every day or are blister packs, where the pills are pushed through. This may also be difficult. If you are on a type of pill where each one is the same, you can ask the pharmacist (or a friend) to put them all into a bottle that has a lid that opens easily. One person told me that she puts a small glob of gum onto a pencil and uses it to pick up a pill and put it into her mouth.

Putting a diaphragm in can also be difficult if you have trouble using your fingers. An inserter (you can get it at the drugstore) can be helpful. You may want your partner to put in your diaphragm for you.

Asthma: The birth control pill does not make asthma worse.

There have been reports of IUD failures (i.e., pregnancy) in people who take steroid medications, such as prednisone. This is unlikely to be a problem with inhaled steroids or with the Mirena IUD, but if you are taking steroids by mouth and have a copper IUD, you should use condoms and foam as well. (Anyone with an IUD should use condoms, as IUDs do not provide protection from sexually transmitted infections.)

Blindness/Visual Impairment: If your decreased vision is caused by a problem with your blood vessels, you may not be able to take the birth control pill. If you are on the Pill, you will need a container that makes it easy to find the next pill (this is especially important with triphasic pills, which have to be taken in the right order). Ask your doctor to show you a variety of containers to choose from. If you are using a diaphragm as birth control, keep the gel with it. If you keep other things in tubes in the same place, smell the gel when you buy it so that you don't get it mixed up with a different one.

Blood Clots (Thromboembolic Disease): You should not be on the Pill if you have had a stroke or any other major problem with clots. If you are on anticoagulants, your doctor may feel it is safe for you to be on the Pill. If the Pill isn't safe for you, she may still want to stop your ovaries from developing eggs, because the development of eggs in your ovaries can lead to hemorrhage. This suppression is done with a nasal spray and is often combined with using vaginal suppositories (big pills you put in your vagina) containing progesterone so that you will continue to have normal periods. This treatment is effective birth control.

Cancer: The birth control pill is safe unless you have a tumor that is considered to be hormone dependent, such as breast cancer or if you have (or ever had) malignant melanoma. Ask your doctor if you have a hormone-dependent tumor before starting on the Pill. If you are on steroids, the copper IUD may be less effective.

Cerebral Palsy: The birth control pill is usually not recommended for anyone who is at increased risk of getting blood clots, and some doctors consider this to include people who spend most of their time in a wheelchair. However, many women who use wheelchairs have been on the Pill. You may find it difficult to insert a diaphragm. Condoms are usually a good method but can be a problem if both partners have difficulty using their hands.

Crohn's Disease and Ulcerative Colitis: Even if your inflammatory bowel disease is stable and not causing problems, the birth control pill should be used only if you can be closely monitored, as the Pill is associated with irritation of the gastrointestinal tract.

If you have malabsorption or other signs of active disease, a form of birth control other than the Pill should be used, as absorption of the hormones in the Pill may be incomplete, leading to a higher risk of pregnancy. Having your colon removed does not interfere with absorption of the Pill, but an ileostomy in which you have part of the small bowel removed or bypassed may interfere with absorption and, in this case, the birth control pill should not be used.

Cystic Fibrosis: There is a theoretical risk that the Pill will make lung secretions thicker, as it increases the thickness of cervical mucus, but in actual use it does not seem to make CF symptoms worse.

Antibiotics (especially rifampicin) can decrease the effectiveness of the Pill, so you should use a backup contraceptive method during cycles in which you are taking antibiotics.

Deafness/Hearing Impairment: All methods of contraception should be safe for you to use.

Diabetes: The birth control pill has been linked to various problems in diabetic women. Many need an increase in insulin dose when on the pill. There is concern that retinopathy may progress more quickly on the Pill and that other blood vessel problems (including stroke and heart attack) may also be increased by being on the Pill. No diabetic with kidney or blood vessel problems should go on the Pill. If you do not have these problems and decide to go on the Pill, you should go on a low-dose pill and have your eyes monitored closely, as well as monitoring your blood sugar carefully. The mini-pill or Depo-Provera are both safe. The Mirena IUD does not affect blood glucose control and is safe and effective to use if you have diabetes.

Hemorrhagic Disorders (hemophilia, von Willebrand disease, etc.): In some people, the birth control pill helps control the heavy periods that can be associated with these conditions. This makes the Pill a good form of birth control for you. There are no reports of the Pill making the condition worse.

The IUD is unsafe if you have a hemorrhagic disorder.

Ileostomy/Colostomy: The Pill may not be completely absorbed before being eliminated if you have an ileostomy, which would make it much less effective. If you really want to try the Pill, use it with condom and foam for a few months. If you are having a normal withdrawal bleed (period) on your days off, and no bleeding in between, then you are probably absorbing an adequate amount.

You may have difficulty using a diaphragm if your rectum was removed, as the shape and position of your vagina may have changed.

Iron Deficiency Anemia: Birth control pills can actually be helpful for this condition. Blood is full of iron, so when you have your period, you are losing iron. When on the Pill, you do not lose as much blood during your period as you otherwise would. Therefore, you don't have to replace as much iron every month.

Because periods tend to be much heavier with a copper IUD, they aren't a good idea if you are iron deficient, but a Mirena is fine.

Kidney Disease: If you do not have high blood pressure, the Pill may be safe for you. It will control your menstrual flow, which will help control the anemia that is common in chronic kidney disease. Your blood pressure needs to be monitored closely, and the Pill must be stopped if your blood pressure goes up. The mini-pill and Depo-Provera are safe.

The copper IUD often causes increased bleeding, which would make anemia worse. The Mirena stops menstrual bleeding, which is highly beneficial if you are anemic. If you have high blood pressure, barrier methods are your best choice.

Liver Disease: The birth control pill affects liver function and should not be used if you have active liver disease or cirrhosis. If you have hepatitis, you should not go on the Pill until your tests of liver function have returned to normal. If you have ever had any liver disease and you go on the Pill, you should have blood tests one to two months after starting it. If they are abnormal, you should stop the Pill. If you and your doctor decide to try an estrogen-containing form of contraception, consider the patch instead of the Pill, as you won't get as high a dose passing through your liver.

Lupus (SLE): Low-dose birth control pills do not seem to make lupus worse. If you have a blood factor that makes getting a clot more likely (lupus anticoagulant or anticardiolipin) you should not go on the Pill, patch or ring. You can use Depo-Provera (but if you have been on steroids a lot, it isn't a great idea, as both can make your bones weaker) or the mini-pill. I have started patients with lupus on the Pill when they had normal blood pressure and no kidney or liver problems, and things have gone well.

If you are taking steroids, a copper IUD may be less effective. If you have a copper IUD and are started on steroids, you should use condoms and foam or another barrier method.

Migraine: Many people who have bad headaches assume they are migraines. If you haven't been diagnosed by a doctor, you should consider it. If your headaches are true migraines and you go on the birth control pill (or other estrogen-containing contraception), your headaches may get worse. If they do, you should go off the Pill. If your headaches are associated with numbness in part of your body, inability to move part of your body, problems seeing or anything else that your doctor has described as a "neurologic" problem, you should use another (non-estrogen) form of birth control. Depo-Provera, an IUD and the mini-pill are probably safe with migraines.

Multiple Sclerosis: There have been reports of MS improving, getting worse and staying the same in people on the birth control pill. Your birth control options are probably as wide as anyone in the general population. The early part of this section outlines these options. If changing pads or inserting tampons is difficult for you, the copper IUD won't be a good choice, as your periods may be much heavier with it.

Neurofibromatosis: Although there is no proof that the Pill can be harmful in this condition, it is felt that you should not use birth control pills if you have neurofibromatosis, as the hormones might cause the lesions to grow. Depo-Provera, an IUD or the mini-pill may be safer.

Since pregnancy makes this condition worse and because of a high incidence of fetal problems, you might want to consider tubal ligation. This must be your decision, and not one that is made for you.

Polycystic Ovarian Disease: If you have this condition, you should be on an estrogen-containing contraceptive to treat your disorder, unless you have a high level of triglycerides (a certain type of fat) in your blood. Products that contain only progestins (like the mini-pill or Depo-Provera) should not be used.

Pulmonary Hypertension: It would be very dangerous for you to go on any birth control that contains estrogen. You should talk with your doctor to see if an IUD insertion would be safe.

Psoriasis: This condition may be worsened by the birth control pill. If the Pill is otherwise the best method for you, you may want to try it and monitor your skin closely. There is a concern that the patch would cause skin problems in the spots you apply it to.

Quadriplegia, Paraplegia, Spina Bifida and Spinal Cord Injury: Some doctors are concerned that people in wheelchairs might be more likely to get blood clots if they take the birth control pill, but others feel that the risk is very small. Many people with spinal cord injury or spina bifida have taken the birth control pill without any problems, but I would recommend that if you want to be on the Pill, Patch or Ring, ask to have the blood test that would show if you are likely to get blood clots.

People who have to catheterize themselves regularly are more likely to have an allergy to latex. If you have a latex allergy, you should not use latex condoms.

If you have an attendant who gives you your medication and you don't want him or her to know you are on the Pill, you can ask a friend or your sexual partner to put them into a bottle for you—but only if you are on the kind of birth control pill that has the same hormone content in each pill. (If they are all the same color, they have the same amount of hormones.) You could also ask a friend to put the Patch on you in an area that your attendant won't see.

The diaphragm or cervical cap requires insertion. An inserter (available at the drugstore) may make it easier to put in a diaphragm. The ring goes inside the vagina, which might be difficult (or impossible) for you to do on your own. A regular sexual partner may be able to learn how to do this for you.

Although the combination of condom and foam is an effective method, you or your partner has to be able to put the condom on and insert the foam.

Scoliosis: If you have severe scoliosis with pelvic involvement, inserting (or being fitted for) a diaphragm may present problems. There may also be difficulty inserting an IUD, but your doctor can advise you about this.

Seizures: As noted in Chapter 5, some seizure medications interact with the birth control pill, increasing the risk of pregnancy. Even with this risk, the Pill is still probably at least as effective as other methods. Valproate does not interact with the birth control pill.

Using a barrier method in addition to the Pill will certainly decrease your chance of pregnancy if you have bleeding in between your periods, a sign that your estrogen levels may be low. Although a small number of women with seizure disorders have had an increase in seizure activity on the Pill, most do not. It is safe for most teens with seizure disorders to be on the birth control pill.

If you decide to have an IUD inserted, you and the doctor doing the procedure should be aware that some people have had grand mal seizures during IUD insertion.

Some women have fewer seizures when on Depo-Provera.

Sickle Cell Anemia and Thalassemia: It used to be thought that people with sickle cell couldn't take the birth control pill, but it is now felt to be safe. Depo-Provera and the mini-pill may actually be helpful in sickle cell disease, as progesterone is thought to stabilize red blood cell membranes.

The copper IUD is not a good choice because of increased blood loss, but the Mirena protects against blood loss.

Some teens with these conditions choose tubal ligation because there are big health risks (to you and the baby) involved with becoming pregnant. As this operation is not easily reversible, you need to think about this option thoroughly before deciding for or against.

Barrier methods (such as the condom and foam combination) are safe with these conditions.

Thyroid Disease: Because the Pill increases something called thyroid binding globulin, your doctor will have to check other things (like free thyroxine) to see if you are getting the right amount of medication if you go on the Pill. Otherwise, you can choose from all the forms of birth control.

Transplantation: If you have had a kidney transplant and do not have high blood pressure, the Pill is probably safe for you. If you have had a liver transplant, most doctors are happier if you use a Mirena, IUD, or the mini-pill, although the Pill is probably safe, particularly the low-dose pills that are available these days. To make things even safer, use the patch, which avoids the effect of hormones being absorbed from the stomach and passing through the liver before going to the rest of the body.

Although the Pill is fairly safe, it can interact with several medications, including some antifungals, antibiotics and antiepileptic medications. The Pill may increase levels of steroids, cyclosporine, tacrolimus and sirolimus, so it is important to get your immunosuppressant levels checked regularly. Many doctors think the Pill should be avoided in the first year after transplant, as other medications and their dosages are changing so much during that time that it can confuse things to add another medication to the mix. However, a pregnancy in the first year could be more of a problem.

Barrier methods are safe and are recommended for young women who have had transplants.

I'm pregnant, and I am trying to decide what to do. I don't feel ready to have a baby, but then I'm not sure how I feel about abortion. I mean, what if my mother had decided to get rid of me? When I tell my doctor, he's going to be mad because I didn't use any birth control. What should I do?

I can't tell you what to do, and neither can anyone else. If you let someone else make this decision for you, you will regret it, I promise.

You have three options at this point. One is to continue the pregnancy and keep that baby. The second is to give up the baby for adoption (this can either be a traditional adoption where you don't know or have any input into who gets the baby, or an "open" adoption where there is some level of connection and choice about this). Third, you can have an abortion, if you are early enough in your pregnancy.

Counting from the first day of your last period, you have 12 weeks to have a first trimester abortion. Very early in the pregnancy, you can have a medical abortion, in which medications cause a miscarriage. These are the safest abortions. In all states in the U.S. and all Canadian provinces, abortions are legal until 12 weeks. Many people are too late in knowing that they are pregnant or in making a decision to have a medical abortion. A first trimester abortion is usually performed by a process called vacuum aspiration, where the contents of your uterus are sucked out with a small tube. Your cervix (the opening from your uterus into your vagina) may be gently opened up in advance by having a device called a laminaria tent inserted into it the day before. It looks like a matchstick, and once it is put in it starts to expand. You may get some cramps when it is inserted.

If you have a first trimester abortion in a clinic, you will probably have a local anesthetic—that is, you will be awake during the procedure. They may give you something to relax you a bit. Abortions performed in a hospital may be done either with a local or a general anesthetic (you will be asleep). A local anesthetic carries less risk, but it might be scary for you to be awake.

Your condition may determine what kind of anesthetic is used. If you have spasms in your legs, a general anesthetic should be used. If you have a heart or lung problem, an anesthetist should assess you and recommend what would be best. It is important that the doctor who performs the abortion know about your condition. If you are on anticoagulants (like warfarin or heparin), you will probably have to be admitted to the hospital.

Second trimester abortions and early third trimester abortions are legal in some places but not in others. They may be performed in a similar way to the first trimester abortions, or may be done by stimulating labor, or by replacing the amniotic fluid around the fetus with salt water.

You have to realize that you aren't going to find a perfect solution to your problem. What you are going to have to find is a solution you can live with, one that seems right to you. Try to make a list of all the good and bad things about each choice. If you find yourself really trying to find more good things to put under one choice, then this is probably the one you should go with. Or you might try flipping a coin and paying attention to what you are hoping it will land on. Check out the last question in this chapter and see if there are dangers to you or your fetus because of your illness or disability. You may want to take this into account.

Don't do anything just because your boyfriend, your parents or your doctor say you should. If you have an abortion you don't really want, you will just get pregnant again. If you have a baby you don't want, you are increasing its risk of being abused or neglected.

See a doctor right away. It may be embarrassing to admit that you didn't protect yourself (or even to tell your doctor that you had sex), but putting this off will only make things worse, will limit your options and perhaps put your health in danger. Make sure you really are pregnant. Discuss all the options available to you and then make your decision. Try to find someone who can give you some emotional support.

Believe it or not, this may be one of your parents. Although parents tend to get mad when their daughters get pregnant, they often (although not always) can get beyond their anger and give much-needed love and support.

I've decided to start having intercourse soon and plan to go on the birth control pill. I've been going to the same doctor since I was little, and I don't want to talk to him about sex. For one thing, I'd be really embarrassed. For another, I'm sure he'd tell my parents. My best friend went to a clinic and got a Pap smear and everything. I thought I'd go there too. Do I need to tell them about my condition?

Yes. Wherever you go to get contraception, you will be asked about illnesses and medications, and it is important to be honest. There might be forms of contraception that are not safe for you. The Pill (oral contraceptives) might make your illness worse or interact to make your medications less effective, or make the levels of medication in your bloodstream too high. Your medication may make the Pill less effective.

I think you should consider telling your doctor that you want to go on the Pill. I know it can be hard to discuss this subject with someone who is old enough to be your father (or grandfather), who is male, who might still think of you as a little girl. But the complex interactions between medications and between medications and your illness mean that it is important for your physician to know what else you are taking. If you end up using a barrier method, it is less important that he know.

Your doctor should not, of course, divulge any information you give him without your permission. This is not to say that there aren't doctors who do this. Try starting a discussion by asking him his policy about confidentiality. Ask him what information he feels he must share with your parents. If he says he tells parents everything, you might want to point out to him that this will stop you and others from discussing things with him that you don't want shared.

I've never had sex with anyone. I am incontinent and wear a diaper. I do also use the bathroom—my incontinence is dribbling that happens in between. I am worried about having sex and what my partner may think.

The first thing to remember is that between female lubrication and male ejaculate (cum), sex is a fairly wet business anyway. So things might not be as difficult as you think.

The second thing is that sex always has to be planned to a certain extent. Unplanned sex carries a high risk of pregnancy and sexually transmitted infection. You are going to have to plan sex more than many people, but that doesn't mean you have to lose enjoyment.

It is hard to know what potential partners will think until you ask them. Some people may be totally turned off. Many will see it as only a minor inconvenience. You should bring it up beforehand. You don't want to end up in bed with someone who is going to be weird about it.

Anyone who is incontinent and has the ability to empty his or her bladder either by going to the bathroom or catheterizing should do so before having sex.

Even if you can do this, you will probably want to have a rubber or plastic sheet on the bed. This is where the planning comes in. This obviously means you can't have sex on the backseat of a car (unless you bring a rubber sheet with you).

If you are going to be at your partner's place, you will have to bring or leave a plastic sheet there. Have a large towel on hand, so you can lie on it after and not have to get up or remake the bed. You may want to have an extra diaper handy so you can slip it on before drifting off to sleep. If you are in a hurry and don't want to stop to put the sheet on, an uncarpeted floor, a shower or the bathtub are all places where you can have sex (and are also used by people without your problem).

> **I am a 14-year-old with arthritis. I hang out mainly with 16- and 17-year-olds. Earlier this year I really wanted to start having sex. I couldn't stand not knowing what it was all about. There was a guy I was really attracted to and I made it pretty clear that I was interested in him. We started having sex on our second date. Some of it has been great—I love the feeling of his body next to mine—but much of the time it just isn't what I expected. I don't think I've had an orgasm, and lots of the time I lie there thinking about what clothes I want to buy. Is this all there is to it?**

There can be many reasons you're not enjoying sex—fatigue from your illness, worries about pregnancy (you don't mention what you are using for birth control), worries about getting caught, being in such a hurry that your body isn't really prepared to have intercourse and others.

What I wonder is if you started having sex before you were ready. You seem to have experienced some sexual feelings and jumped right into intercourse. It is often a good idea to explore your sexuality at a somewhat slower pace—fantasizing what you would like with someone else, masturbating to discover what stimulates you and what doesn't, and meeting someone you are attracted to and letting the sexual tension build between you. Communication is an essential part of good sex, and it is unlikely that you established this on one date.

You seem to have made a decision to become sexually active and to have pursued this, as opposed to developing a relationship, becoming more and more sexual and then deciding to have sex. You state that one of your main drives was curiosity. Was it perhaps also a feeling of wanting to be "normal," to show (to yourself and to others) that there is nothing different about you, even though you have arthritis? This is not uncommon in people who feel there is something different about them. Most teens want to be like their friends and to do things that show they aren't kids anymore.

Whatever your reasons, you now seem to feel stuck with a sexual relationship that doesn't make you happy. You need to understand that just because you have started having intercourse does not mean you have to continue. Your boyfriend may be feeling as bored with the sex part of your relationship as you are. But even if he isn't, I think it is time for you to take a vacation from sex.

Talk to your boyfriend and explain that you feel you two have missed out on some of the earlier stages of a relationship by starting to have sex right at the beginning. Suggest to him that you would like to start over, going out, talking, holding hands, hugging. Let him know that you can't guarantee you will want to start having sex again. Spend some time by yourself thinking about what you want out of a relationship. You can use this time to get to know and value yourself better too.

What if he says he doesn't want to see you if you won't have sex? You'll have to make a decision about what to do, but it seems to me that if he is interested in you as a person, he'll agree, and if he doesn't really care about you as a person, then you shouldn't be having sex with him.

I was born with bladder extrophy and had lots of surgery on my belly and penis. The doctor keeps referring to my penis as a "great repair." Unless there are tons of guys out there with penises that look like short cauliflowers, he's lying. How am I ever going to have sex? Even if I can physically do it, won't my scars and my weird-looking penis scare girls off?

First, let me address the question of whether your doctor is lying. I suspect that you and he have very different definitions of a "great repair." His standard for a good repair might be the ability to pee or something like that. He's probably never thought of how he would feel if his penis looked like yours. There is a likelihood that he is comparing your penis to what it looked like when you were born. You, of course, can't remember this. He may have taken pictures at the time, which you might want to ask to see. It may give you a better idea of where he's coming from.

When thinking about sex, keep in mind the following points. (1) When women are asked what is physically most important to them in an intimate relationship, the response from many is cuddling, hugging and kissing. (2) Men and women do many things in bed together that do not involve a penis in the vagina. (3) Many of the aforementioned things can lead to orgasm. (4) Only a few women think the size of a man's penis is important. (5) You are probably right that you are going to experience some difficulties, but you should be able to get around them because of points 1 to 4.

The hardest thing for you is going to be explaining to a potential partner what your problem is. The timing is tricky (not too early in the relationship, nor five minutes before you are going to take your clothes off). You will probably feel somewhat embarrassed, which will likely make you less articulate. Early on in a relationship, you may want to mention that you have had surgery several times. As the two of you get closer, you can talk about how you feel about your abdominal scars and worries you may have about how they affect your attractiveness. Before you talk to her about your penis, practice what you are going to say, either with a friend who already knows or in front of your mirror. Don't just not say anything. You know what you are going to see every time you look at your penis, and you still don't feel great about it. If she sees it without any foreknowledge, she is likely to have a strong reaction that will make you feel terrible and make her feel guilty afterward.

You may have difficulty at first finding someone who is understanding about this and who feels comfortable enough about her own sexuality to be comfortable with your differences. But as people grow older and mature (and many do mature), they look more and more for a sexual partner who has attractive qualities that are not just physical.

There are many girls who would prefer to perform oral sex on someone with a smaller penis, so having a penis that is smaller than average might have a distinct advantage.

You and your partner will need to feel very comfortable with each other before you attempt penetrative sex (if this is what the two of you decide you want). Explore each other's bodies, discover what she likes, let her find out what you like. If you do have intercourse, you might want to start with you on your back with her on top of you.

One problem you are almost sure to run into is finding a condom that fits. Buy a few different brands and try them on while you are masturbating. They do stretch, so you will be able to get it on over any bulges, but your penis may not be long enough to hold one on. There are a few snugger-fit condoms available. If you live in a place that has a condom store or a good sex-toy store, this is where to look. Also guys roll the condom down and pull it behind their scrotum to hold it on, but I don't know if this would work for everyone.

If you and your partner decide to try penetration, you'll want to experiment with positions, but it is likely you'll have the most success with her on top.

I don't know if you will be successful with penetration, but I do know that with or without it, you have the potential for a satisfying sexual life.

It's easy to say that an able-bodied guy is going to want to have sex with me. How is he going to know what will feel good for me? How will I know what he wants—I've never had a perfect body.

Well, to start with, he's never had a perfect body either. I can guarantee you that anyone you go out with will have spent hours worrying about his body—his height, his hair, his skin, his muscles, his teeth, whatever.

Second, even if you had bodies that were matched in their disability, you still wouldn't have a body like his, because he's male and you're female. This is a much bigger difference than any others you may have.

Of course, he's not going to know what you want, and you won't know what he wants. You'll both be able to make some guesses, but don't assume they are right. He may be a bit shyer about making these guesses because he may have picked up on your attitude that there is something about you that is essentially different from other girls.

What the two of you will have to do is what anyone—male, female, gay, straight, disabled or not—has to do to have good sex. The first thing is to have respect for your partner. This is an experience you are sharing, not something one person does to the other. Part of this respect is to have sex with a person because it is what you really want, with that particular person, not for other reasons like wanting to know what sex is like, wanting to get it over with, wanting to make someone else jealous.

The second thing is to talk. This can be hard. We aren't used to talking about sex. We aren't taught to ask for what we want. Never pretend to like something that you feel uncomfortable about. Never assume that he does or doesn't want to do something with you. Check it out. Talking about sex doesn't have to be clinical. It can be a very exciting interaction.

Lastly, don't expect things to be perfect all the time. Not every idea works. You don't always feel like doing whatever it was you enjoyed the last time. Give yourselves time to learn about each other.

Someone told me that guys with sickle cell can get a hard-on that doesn't go away and really hurts. Now I'm scared to masturbate. Is this true, or was he just trying to scare me?

Boys and men with sickle cell can get something called priapism, an erection that won't go away. (It's like having a sickle cell crisis in your penis.) Boys younger than 12 hardly ever have this happen to them, but a study of Jamaican adult men with sickle cell showed that half of them had had this problem at least once.

You get an erection when big spaces in your penis fill with blood. If your blood cells are in a sickle form, the blood can have a hard time getting out again.

This problem is just as likely to occur with the erection you get in the morning as it is with masturbation or other sexual activity, so worries about it are no reason to avoid sexual activity.

There is really nothing you can do to prevent it from happening. Someone did a study giving men a drug to stop erections to prevent this, but this seems somewhat extreme to me.

If you get an erection that doesn't go away after you have an orgasm, or a morning erection that doesn't go away after the usual time, you need to see your doctor right away. Yes, it may be embarrassing, but it is important not to let this go on too long. If you go for 24 hours without medical treatment to make it better, you have a high chance of not being able to have erections again. Your doctor will probably start by giving you a transfusion and painkillers, but if it doesn't get better, a surgeon will remove the blood with a needle.

It may be hard not to worry about this, but if you can manage to put it out of your mind, your life will be easier.

Ever since an accident three years ago (when I was 13), I have been quadriplegic. I have spent most of the time in a rehab hospital and will be moving out soon. My boyfriend and I are looking for an apartment. I am on the Pill but I plan to go off soon so that I can be pregnant by the time we move in together. My boyfriend is very supportive and I know things will work out. Are there any special things I should be concerned about?

There is nothing about being quadriplegic that means you can't get pregnant, have a child and be a good parent. Obviously, you will need help in physically caring for your child, but you should be able to breastfeed. Talking with your child and being a warm loving parent are more important than getting to be the person who changes the diapers (although you may be able to do this too). You should, however, talk to your doctor about such things as whether any of your medications could harm a growing fetus.

There are some special considerations involved with being 16 and a parent. A strong relationship between parents is very important. This doesn't just mean being in love. It means developing strong patterns of communication that will carry you through times of no sleep and very reduced romantic interchanges. Parenting a young child often means putting your own personal development on hold while attending to your child's development.

Have you really thought about why you want to have a child at this point in your life? Are you maybe trying to prove to the world (or some specific people in it) that you are "normal?" Is this a way to show that you are not a kid anymore? If you are looking for a relationship in which you will always be loved, it is important to remember that your child will not always act loving toward you. You could easily have a baby who cries all day and all night.

Part of normal development for young children is to separate from their parents, to form a sense of themselves as people in their own right, and one of the ways they do this is through "oppositional behavior"—doing the opposite of what the parent wants them to. You can be sure your child will not always do what you want as he or she begins to become a unique individual, and times like this are very trying.

What is your rush, anyway? You are likely to be fertile for the next 25 years. Why not spend a year learning to live with your boyfriend, and see how things go? Go out to movies and have fun. One of the things that made losing my social life bearable when I had small children was knowing that I already had a few years of going on vacation, eating in restaurants, seeing movies and having time for friends. Think carefully of any reasons that you have for becoming pregnant this year instead of next year. Will you get more money from welfare? It doesn't cover the extra cost of having a kid. To stop your boyfriend from leaving you if you have his child? Think again. Many guys can't handle the responsibility and hassle of having a baby and leave when they might have stayed if a third person hadn't been added to the relationship.

Have you tried practicing some parenting? See if a friend will "lend" you and your boyfriend her baby or toddler for an afternoon or evening. The two of you should do everything the baby needs. This will give you some useful experience, and you'll be able to see how your boyfriend interacts with a child.

Of course, I'm not saying you'll be a terrible parent. If you decide to get pregnant soon, I am sure you will work hard to do your best, and your best will probably be pretty good. The emotional cost may be very high, though. If waiting a year or two can make it an easier job, why not do this?

Whenever you decide to get pregnant, I would strongly advise you to have a midwife as one of your caregivers. Midwives provide incredible support and are very knowledgeable. Your midwife will help you throughout your pregnancy, labor and delivery and in the first weeks of your child's life. She can help you get in touch with other people who are parenting from wheelchairs.

This is the biggest decision you will ever make. Once you have a child, you will always be a mother. Give it careful thought and then stick to whatever you feel is the right decision for you.

I was in the hospital last week. The night before I went home, my girlfriend came to visit. After she left, my nurse came in and did my vital signs and said goodnight. For once I was in a private room, and when the nurse left I closed the door and started to jerk off. All of a sudden the nurse came back in. She turned around and left. I was so embarrassed. I know I should have gone out and apologized, but I just couldn't.

No, you shouldn't. She should have waited a reasonable amount of time, knocked on the door, and apologized for walking in on you without knocking. A closed door is a symbol in our culture, one that says, "I want privacy." It is not rude to masturbate in private. Your room should have been private once you shut the door.

Hopefully this nurse has learned her lesson and will never walk in on anyone again. There are still other health care professionals who will, however, and without a dramatic incident like this, they may not ever change their behavior.

Next time you go to the hospital, you could take a sign with you that says "Please knock" and post it on your door. It may not always work, and you may worry that everyone will think you are always masturbating, even when you are just reading or watching TV with the door shut.

Even bathrooms aren't always safe, although people are much more likely to knock. They also aren't the most pleasant places to express your sexuality.

I have always wanted to have children. I baby-sit frequently and have just started an Early Childhood Education course. I love having children in my life and would like some of my own. My boyfriend and I are getting married soon, and when I talk about having kids he gets scared and says maybe it won't be healthy for me. I think he is also worried that we will have a child with the same problem I have. How can I get more information?

You are asking several questions here. Will pregnancy affect your health? Will your state of health affect your pregnancy? What are the chances your child will have the same condition as you have? In addition, many teens with a chronic illness or disability wonder if they can become pregnant or get someone pregnant. The easy answer to all these questions is that you and your boyfriend should talk with your doctor about this. Consider spending some time figuring out what all your questions are before you go. You can write them down and take them with you to the appointment so you don't forget something important. You may want to leave enough space on the paper to write down the answers.

In preparation, here is some general information about pregnancy and illness or disability, and specific information regarding certain conditions. Remember that everyone is different, so even if I say there is a high (or low) risk of something, you should still talk with your doctor. Your doctor can also find out if any of your medications could harm a fetus in any way. This concern should be researched well in advance, as your doctor may have to find some alternative medications for you that might have to be switched before you get pregnant. Some people will find out in a discussion like this that it would be very unsafe for them to have a child, or that it is impossible to get pregnant. This information is very difficult to receive. You and your boyfriend may feel devastated. Many people find it helps to talk with other people in the same situation. Most cities have support groups for people who want to have children and can't get pregnant. If your doctor doesn't know of one, a clinic that does assessments for infertility should, so try calling there.

There is the potential that your condition may worsen because of pregnancy and delivery. Changes in your health may be temporary or permanent, and can be minor or severe.

Although an occasional, small amount of alcohol is probably safe in pregnancy, higher levels can lead to severe problems in the child. Other street drugs (such as amphetamines and cocaine) can also lead to problems and should be avoided in pregnancy. If you are trying to get pregnant, you should assume that you are pregnant when making decisions about drinking or taking drugs.

Being seriously ill can affect fertility temporarily. Women with chronic illness often notice that they miss their period when they are very sick. Illness is less likely to affect male fertility.

Many women miss their period (and are probably not fertile) when on high-dose steroids. Although many doctors think that this is due to how sick you have to be to be on these high doses, this could also be related to the steroids.

Some conditions are genetic—that is, they can be passed on through your genes to your children and subsequent generations. Being born with something doesn't necessarily make it genetic, and some genetic conditions show up later in life. You may need to ask your doctor if your condition is genetic. There are different kinds of genetic inheritance. All of our genes are paired—we get one of each type from each parent. Every time you get pregnant, your fetus gets half of your genes (one from each pair) and half of your partner's genes, resulting in a full set of genes.

A dominant gene is one that overpowers the other gene in the pair. For example, the gene for brown eyes is dominant over the gene for blue eyes. If you get a brown-eyed gene from one parent and a blue-eyed gene from the other, you'll have brown eyes. If your condition is caused by a dominant gene, you likely have one gene that codes for the condition, while the other one in the pair doesn't. If this is the case, every time you release an egg (potentially leading to pregnancy), it has a 50% chance of having either the gene for the condition or the more common gene that does not cause the condition. If your partner has the same dominant gene, then there is a 75% chance each time that the fetus will have that gene (or two of them) and therefore your condition. With a number of conditions, having two copies of the gene will result in a miscarriage.

A recessive gene is one that causes the disability or illness only if matched with another recessive gene. So if your partner doesn't have your condition and doesn't carry the gene, all your children will be carriers (meaning they can pass the gene along to their kids) but none will have the disease. If your partner carries the gene (and doctors can now test for some but not all genes), each of your children has a 50% chance of either having the disease or being a carrier. If your partner has the same condition, then all your children will have the condition.

There is a gene pair that determines your sex. Girls and women have two X genes, and boys and men have an X and a Y gene, so gender is determined by the father, who donates either an X (the baby will be a girl) or a Y (the baby will be a boy). Some conditions are X-linked, that is, they are carried on an X gene and are dominant over a Y gene, but not over a "normal" X gene. These conditions are therefore much more common in boys (who get the disease with one affected X) but can occur in girls who have two X genes that code for the condition. Hemophilia is the most well known of these conditions. So, if you are a male with an X-linked condition, your daughters will all carry the gene but will not be affected by the condition unless your partner also carries the gene. Your sons will not get the gene from you, as you give them your Y gene. Boys get X-linked conditions from their mothers only, who usually carry the gene without knowing it.

There are also conditions where there is a genetic predisposition—that is, they run in families but don't follow strict rules of inheritance. This may be because a combination of genes code for the disease, or because other factors in the environment or within your body lead to the condition when combined with the gene. If you have one of these conditions, your children will have a higher chance of getting it than the general population, but this may not be a huge risk. For example, a disease may be present in 4% of the general population, in 6% of children with one affected parent and in 10% of children with two parents who have the condition.

If you have a genetic condition, you need to think about the possibility of raising a child with the same condition you have. Whatever the chance, talk with your boyfriend about how you feel. There is no right approach. It may be clear to you that you are happy with your life, that your condition has been only a minor inconvenience and that you will have no difficulties if your child has your condition. On the other hand, you may feel that you have suffered a great deal and do not want your child to suffer in the same way. Take these feelings and combine them with what you know about your child's chances of having your condition, about the possibility of prenatal diagnosis (having the fetus tested to see if it will have your condition) and your feelings about abortion and adoption, and you will eventually come up with a decision that suits you and your boyfriend.

For some reason, people often feel they have the right to make comments about very personal things in other people's lives, so don't be surprised if you hear from some of these busybodies about your decision. You may get this no matter what you decide. You do not have to justify yourself to these people. Tell them it was a personal decision and none of their business.

About one in five pregnancies ends in a miscarriage or fetal death. Many women who have no health problems have miscarriages. If you lose a pregnancy, do not assume that it is because of your other condition. It may be, but there is a very good chance that it is unconnected.

If you are unable to have intercourse, artificial insemination may be a possibility. You can try this yourself for a few months before getting involved with a fertility clinic. The woman needs to figure out when she is ovulating. There are several ways to do this, including taking your temperature in the morning before you get up and charting it, and observing your cervical mucus. Natural family planning courses offered by Catholic agencies are often a good way to learn how to do this. There are also urine tests that can be bought at the drugstore without a prescription, but they tend to be expensive. On the day the woman ovulates (or even the day before, the day of and the day after), the man ejaculates into a jar (if he has difficulty using his hands, he may need someone to hold the jar) and then the semen is squirted into the vagina with a syringe (no needle!). Lie down for about half an hour afterward. If neither you nor your partner can manipulate the syringe, you will need help. If the male cannot ejaculate or knows that he does not have enough sperm in his semen to get a woman pregnant, another possibility is artificial insemination by donor semen, usually performed in a clinic.

I have been told that the book *Mother to Be: A Guide to Pregnancy and Birth for Women with Disabilities* by Judith Rogers and Molleen Matsumura is very good. You may want to see if your library carries it.

The following information is about specific conditions (listed alphabetically), fertility and pregnancy. Remember that there may be new information that has become available since the publication of this book, and that solutions may have been found for problems I point out, so use what I have provided as a starting point for your discussion with your doctor, and don't make any final decisions based just on this information. Pregnancies in the general population result in a 4% to 6% rate of what are called congenital anomalies (something different about a newborn physically or in the way their body works) so I can't promise anyone that her child will be born totally healthy.

Arthritis: Some people with arthritis find that their health improves while they are pregnant. Some get sicker after the baby is born. The delivery may be more difficult if your hips are affected by arthritis.

Your ability to get pregnant or get your partner pregnant should not be affected by your condition.

Asthma: Asthma has not been shown to affect fertility in either males or females. Women with asthma report a variety of effects during pregnancy—no change, more attacks, fewer attacks. Your medications are unlikely to affect the child, but you should speak with your doctor. Asthma does tend to run in families, so your children are at increased risk of having this problem.

Blindness/Visual Impairment: Your ability to get pregnant (or to get your partner pregnant), or to be pregnant and have the baby is the same as for the general population.

There are many causes of visual impairment and blindness. Your doctor should be able to tell you if there is a chance that you will pass this on to your children.

Cancer: Radiation treatments can lead to infertility in both males and females, especially if the ovaries or testicles were in the radiation field. If you are unable to have periods without medication, it is quite likely that your ovaries are not working. Males can have a test done to measure the sperm count (number of sperm in your semen). If the count is low, a counselor or doctor at an infertility program will talk with you about options such as artificial insemination with donor semen.

If you have radiation treatments in the first month of pregnancy, there can be severe effects on the fetus. Chemotherapy in the first three months of pregnancy can also cause a miscarriage or problems for the fetus. If possible, it is recommended that you wait at least one year after having chemotherapy or radiation before getting pregnant. Males can ask their doctors how long to wait before fathering a child, which will relate to how long it will take to clear the medication from your system.

Unless you have a hormone-dependent tumor, a pregnancy should not make your cancer worse or make you go out of remission.

Some tumors that very young children get are passed on in families from either males or females, so if you had cancer when you were very young, check with your doctor about the likelihood of your child being affected.

Cerebral Palsy: Whether you are male or female, if you are able to have intercourse, your fertility will probably not be affected by your condition. If you are unable to have intercourse, then artificial insemination with your or your partner's semen can be done. If spasms are a problem for the pregnant woman, the delivery may be difficult and a cesarean section may be needed.

CP is not genetic, so you cannot pass it on to your children, although they have the same chance of having CP as any other child.

As there are various forms of this condition, you should talk with your doctor before getting pregnant. Chances of passing it on to your children are small.

Congenital Adrenal Hyperplasia: If you take your medication regularly, then you have a good chance of getting pregnant or getting someone pregnant. However, if you don't take your medications as directed, you may run into problems. Women who have the salt-losing form of the disease are more likely to have a hard time getting pregnant. Women who can't (or don't want to) have intercourse can have artificial insemination.

Men with CAH who don't take their meds all the time have an increased chance of getting a tumor in or near the testicle that can stop sperm from getting out of the testicle. This can usually be treated without an operation, but if an operation is needed, it can be done without removing the testicle.

As there are various forms of this problem, you should talk with your doctor before getting pregnant. Chances of passing it on to your children are small. A genetics counselor can help you understand the chances of your child having CAH and the genetics of your condition.

Crohn's Disease and Ulcerative Colitis: Other than when women don't have their period because they are very ill, neither of these inflammatory bowel diseases affect fertility. If your disease has been under control for a year or more, you will probably have a normal pregnancy and have a normal healthy child.

There seems to be a genetic predisposition to these diseases, so your children have a slightly increased risk of getting your illness.

Cystic Fibrosis: If you are male, there is a strong chance that you cannot get a woman pregnant without help. A fertility specialist can test your sperm count. Men with CF make sperm, but the sperm can't make their way into the semen. There are techniques for extracting sperm and then using them to fertilize the woman's eggs. Another option is artificial insemination by donor sperm. (It isn't sperm that makes you a dad, it's parenting.) If you are female, you can probably get pregnant, depending on how sick you are. Because of thick cervical mucus, it may be harder to get pregnant, but there are techniques to improve the chance of pregnancy.

Cystic fibrosis is caused by a recessive gene, so your children each have a 50% chance of having CF if your partner is a carrier, and close to none if he or she isn't.

If your weight is normal for your height, your chest X-ray is close to normal and you have pretty good pulmonary function, you are likely to have a good pregnancy and a healthy baby. However, if you are underweight, have an abnormal chest X-ray or poor pulmonary function, you are taking a big risk of getting sicker or even dying and of having a baby who is small, sick or dies. Any pregnancy should be carefully planned with your doctor.

Deafness/Hearing Impairment: If you are female, your ability to get pregnant, be pregnant and have a healthy baby will not be affected; a male's ability to get someone pregnant is also not affected by his condition.

Deafness can be caused by many things. If you became deaf from an infection or medications, you cannot pass it on to your children. If you were born deaf, it might be genetic. Talk with your doctor about the chance of passing it on.

Diabetes: The better your control of your diabetes, the more likely you are to get pregnant and to have a healthy pregnancy and child. Your baby may be larger than other babies. If you are planning to have children, you should consider having them when you are fairly young (between 18 and 30), as you should not get pregnant if you have vascular complications, which come with age. If your control of your diabetes is poor, especially in the first few months of pregnancy, you have an increased chance of having a baby with a heart problem.

Children of diabetic fathers are more likely to be diabetic (about 7% become diabetic) than children of diabetic mothers (about 4%). The reason for this is not known.

Diabetic men with vascular complications may have decreased fertility.

Heart Disease: The most common heart problems are those that allow blood to flow from the left side of the heart to the right side (the wrong way). These conditions are most often because of holes in the wall that separates heart chambers but can also be from other causes. If this is your problem, you have a higher than average chance of having a child who also has this problem, but you are still likely to have a child with no heart problem. If your heart is functioning well, it is probably safe for you to be pregnant and have a child, but you should talk to your doctor.

If you have an outflow obstruction such as pulmonary or aortic stenosis or coarctation of the aorta, and you have fairly good heart function, you will probably have a living, normal-weight baby. There is about a one-in-five chance that a child who has one parent with one of these types of heart problem will also have a heart problem.

If you have a low level of oxygen in your blood (if you have cyanosis), you have a high chance of having trouble carrying a pregnancy. You are more likely to have a child who is small, who is premature or who will die during your pregnancy or shortly after. This is because the fetus, like you, is not getting enough oxygen. If you used to be cyanotic and this has been corrected, your chance of having a living, normal-weight baby is close to what anyone else would have.

If you have pulmonary hypertension, it can be quite risky for you to be pregnant. See the PH section below.

Iron Deficiency Anemia: You should try to get this under control before getting pregnant, as your body will be supplying all the fetus's iron needs. Since iron supplements and pregnancy are both constipating, you will need a strategy to get around this, like taking your iron with a glass of prune juice, getting more iron in your diet and less from supplements, or trying different preparations.

Iron deficiency is not an inherited condition.

Kidney Disease: If you have severe kidney disease but are not yet on dialysis, you may have a hard time getting and staying pregnant. Once on dialysis, your fertility will improve. Unless you have high blood pressure that cannot be controlled, the pregnancy should not have an effect on your health. You will have a higher chance of miscarriage or stillbirth, but women on dialysis have had normal, healthy children. If you have a transplant, you should wait at least one year before getting pregnant. It is possible that your new kidney will not work as well as a result of a pregnancy, and there may be a risk to the fetus from your immunosuppressive medication.

Not as much is known about fertility in men with kidney disease, but it is likely that fertility is somewhat decreased when you are in renal failure but not on dialysis, but that it improves on dialysis.

Some forms of kidney disease are genetic, but not all. Your doctor should be able to talk with you about the chance of passing on your condition to your children.

Lupus (SLE): About a third of women with lupus have no change in their condition while pregnant, a third get worse and a third improve. About 10% of women with lupus have some permanent worsening in their kidney function during pregnancy. Some babies are born with problems with their heart rhythm, which can be severe. Your baby should be closely monitored during and after birth.

Men with lupus who have been treated with IV cyclophosphamide have a high risk of fertility problems. Some doctors recommend that men who will get this medication intravenously donate sperm for freezing before treatment, but I have not heard of this being offered to teens.

MRKH: With this condition, you do not have a uterus and so cannot be pregnant. However, you have ovaries, so it is possible to have eggs removed and fertilized in a lab (in vitro fertilization), then implanted in a surrogate mother.

Multiple Sclerosis (MS): MS can affect fertility in both men and women. Women with MS who become pregnant may have a normal pregnancy, although in some cases you may find that it makes your condition worse. Spasms may make the delivery difficult.

Your children probably have about a 1-in-100 chance of getting MS at some point. If you are thinking of having a child, you may wish to see a geneticist to get the latest figures on this risk.

Muscular Dystrophy (MD): With either males or females, back or leg problems may make intercourse difficult; if so, you may need to use artificial insemination. Otherwise, your fertility should not be affected by your condition. Delivery may be complicated by back and hip problems, and bearing down (to push the baby out) may be difficult.

As there is more than one kind of MD, you should talk to your doctor about the chance of passing on your condition to your baby.

Neurofibromatosis: Pregnancy can lead to increased health problems, including the development of high blood pressure. There is also a higher than usual chance of miscarriage and stillbirth.

This condition is genetic, passed on by a dominant gene, so you have a 50% chance of passing this on to each child you have.

Ostomy: If your rectum or bladder has been removed, your uterus may change position, making it more difficult to get pregnant. Also, having a stoma pins down your intestine or ureters in one place, whereas normally they have a bit of potential movement and can get out of the way of the uterus. Talk to your doctor to see if, in your case, the pressure of your growing uterus will cause any problems.

Following urostomy and colostomy, many men have retrograde ejaculation, which occurs when the semen goes backwards instead of out the urethra. The semen ends up in the bladder, interfering with fertility. If you do ejaculate backwards, you can empty your bladder before sex, then empty the sperm out of the bladder after and use it for artificial insemination. You can try this yourself, using a syringe that has no needle to squirt the semen into your partner's vagina around the time of ovulation.

People have ostomies for a wide variety of reasons, a few because of a genetic disorder. Talk to your doctor to see if you can pass on your condition to your child.

Ovaries that don't work: If you have had your ovaries removed, have lost the function of your ovaries because of chemotherapy or radiation, or were born without any, you do not have eggs (ova) to create a child. If you have a uterus, it may be possible to have in vitro fertilization, using an egg donated by a family member or an unrelated donor. This technique is very expensive.

If you do have in vitro fertilization, your children will not inherit your condition. They will get half their genes from the donor and half from your partner.

Pulmonary Hypertension: Pregnancy is quite risky with PH, but there have been women who have had successful pregnancies with PH. If you are considering a pregnancy, you need to talk with your doctor about your pressures and whether they are low enough for you to survive a pregnancy. If it seems like a possibility, your next step is to go to a high-risk obstetrician who has experience with PH and plan carefully.

Seizures: About half of pregnant women have no change in how many seizures they get when pregnant. About 40% get more seizures, and 10% have fewer. There is no way to predict which group you will be in. Your disorder should not affect the health of your child. Some seizure medications can cause problems to the fetus, so make sure you talk with your doctor before getting pregnant. If you become pregnant accidentally, see a doctor immediately.

Seizures do not have an effect on female or male fertility.

Sickle Cell Anemia: You will probably have no difficulty in getting pregnant (or getting someone pregnant), but pregnancy can be difficult. It is likely that you will experience more sickle cell crises, and there is an increased risk of blood clots to the lungs or kidneys, lung infections and stroke. It is important to talk with your doctor before planning a pregnancy, or before deciding to continue an unplanned one.

Sickle cell is passed on by a recessive gene, so if your partner also has the disease, all your children will have it. If your partner is a carrier (this can be determined by a simple blood test), each child has a 50% chance of having the disease. If your partner is not a carrier, none of your children will have it, but they will all be carriers.

Spina Bifida and Spinal Cord Injuries: If you are female, your fertility should not be affected by your condition. If intercourse is difficult, artificial insemination can be done. If you have abnormalities of your pelvic bones, you may have some problems carrying the baby the full nine months. Spasticity can make delivery more difficult, leading to an increased chance of having a cesarean section.

If you are male, your fertility will be affected if you do not ejaculate or if you ejaculate backwards into your bladder. Other than this, you should be fertile. If you do ejaculate backwards, you can empty your bladder before sex, then empty the sperm out of the bladder after and use it for artificial insemination. You can try this yourself, using a syringe that has no needle to squirt the semen into your partner's vagina around the time of ovulation.

There is a genetic predisposition to neural tube defects (spina bifida is one of these). Your doctor will probably recommend that you start taking folic acid (a B vitamin) for several months before you get pregnant and during pregnancy, as this decreases the chance that your baby will have a neural tube defect. Neural tube defects can often be diagnosed by ultrasound during pregnancy.

Thalassemia: If you have had chelation therapy from a young age and have stuck with it, chances are, male or female, you are fertile, although it may be harder for you to get pregnant than someone who doesn't have thalassemia. If you are not having regular periods, you probably have a buildup of iron in your pituitary gland and it is unlikely that you can get pregnant. If you are on Desferol, most doctors advise going off it for the first three months of pregnancy. If you have had regular chelation therapy, it is probably safe for you to be off it for nine months while you are pregnant, but you will want to make this decision with your doctor. Exjade has been shown to be safe in rat pregnancies, but there isn't any good data on real people, so the advice is to go off it when you get pregnant.

Thalassemia is passed on through a recessive gene. If your partner also has thalassemia, all your children will have it. If your partner is a carrier, each child has a 50% chance of being thalassemic—any who aren't will be carriers. If your partner isn't a carrier, none will have the disease, but all will be carriers.

Thyroid Disease: If you are on thyroid replacement medication, it is important that you take it during pregnancy. If you don't, you have a high chance of either losing the baby or having a major pregnancy complication.

Antithyroid medications may pose a threat to your fetus, so if you are taking these drugs and get pregnant, talk to your doctor immediately.

SEX. CONTRACEPTION. PREGNANCY. A lot to think about. My advice: Start with sexual fantasy, move to sex with another person only when you are comfortable doing so and if you are having heterosexual intercourse, use contraception until you decide you want to be a parent and have a clear plan for how that will work.

Recreation

RECREATION IS MORE than just going to gym class. It is all those things in life that we do for enjoyment. It includes being with friends, exercising and creating things. Recreation is an important part of growing up. It is not something that can be dispensed with when "more important" things come up. Yes, having a chronic condition may sometimes cut into your recreational time. But time for what you enjoy should not always be the first sacrifice. Even when you are in the hospital, you should make sure you do something for yourself every day, even if it is just talking to a friend on the phone.

I have included some questions about driving in this chapter. Driving is important for non-recreational activities such as work and education, but it plays a big part in adolescent social life, and that is why I have made the topic part of this chapter.

> **I am a 15-year-old with spina bifida. I wear leg braces and use crutches. My mother thinks I should participate only in individual sports because I'll get hurt if I'm playing with other people. As much as I like to swim, I get bored swimming on my own and feel left out of things at school. I'm thinking of threatening to switch to scuba diving. Do you think this will work?**

Work, as in grounding you for the rest of your life? Yes, it might. I think you'd be wiser to have some well organized arguments before you talk with her.

The first thing to know is that the biggest danger of most team sports is that some coaches do not demand an adequate warm-up before playing. It is essential that all players have at least 10 minutes of slow, smooth stretching to get their muscles ready for exercise. Many sports injuries are the result of poor warm-up. Avoid bending your head backwards during warm-up.

Do you know what sport you want to play? If so, talk to the coach and see if he or she has any concerns. Get in touch with your country's Paralympic Committee (see Appendix 2 for contact information) and ask if there is an organization for that sport. If there is, get any information it has or see if there is an athlete in your area you could talk with.

Having got all the information you can, go back to your mother and tell her what you want to do. Explain the risks of not being active, and tell her that you are losing your interest in solitary sports. Assure her that you will always do a good warm-up (and do it). If this doesn't convince her, get your doctor on your side.

Don't give up your swimming. It is a great sport and will keep you in good shape year round.

I've always enjoyed hanging out with my friends. We'd go to a mall or go downtown and just walk around, looking in windows and talking. We'd get wherever we were going on public transport. Now that I have Crohn's disease, I never know when I'm going to need a bathroom, and when I need it, I need it soon. I can't figure out how to find bathrooms when I'm out. My friends are starting to think I don't like them anymore because I just go

home after school. Even my parents, who tend to be overprotective, are nagging me to get out more. I finally told my best friend why I wasn't going out and she agreed that it would be difficult to find bathrooms. Is there any answer to this?

I talked to a group of teens with Crohn's disease who seemed to be living pretty active lives and asked what they do about it.

They suggested that you scout out the malls you go to. They all have public bathrooms but they can be hard to find when you are in a hurry. Go with your best friend (or even your mother) and ask at the information desk where the bathrooms are. They might have a map. Then go to these locations to be sure you can find the bathrooms. Note nearby landmarks (names of stores, fountains, etc.). If there is a food area at the mall, there is usually a bathroom nearby.

Large restaurants and chain fast-food places are easier to go into than smaller restaurants. People in smaller restaurants can be awful about access to bathrooms. If there is a downtown area where you often go, ask one of your parents to help you check out the hotels in the area. They all have bathrooms, and you just have to walk in as if you know what you're doing. It helps to have found the bathrooms in advance and to feel that you know your way around a bit.

Do an Internet search for "public restrooms" and name the city or neighborhood. You will often be taken to a travel site, as it is one of the things that tourists want to find out about.

If you are in a big city, subway stations sometimes have public bathrooms. Again, they are not easy to find, so check it out in advance.

Always have toilet paper or tissues with you. This is easier if you are a girl and carry a purse, but girls and guys can always stuff some into a pocket or take a backpack. If you have concerns that you might not make it in time, you can wear a "light days" type menstrual pad and carry a couple of extras. Even guys can do this—they are thin and self-adhesive—and you can get your mother to buy them for you.

What do you say to your friends when you have to stop frequently? You can be truthful and say that you have to go to the bathroom often. If you aren't comfortable with everyone knowing but have a few friends you trust, ask them to take turns saying they have to go to the bathroom when you signal them, then offer to go with them. If you don't want to tell anyone, you'll have to go with the usual random excuses ("I have to get something for my mother. I'll meet you guys soon," "I dropped my bag [book, whatever]. I'll just run back and meet you in front of…")

The worst thing to do would be to sit around your house after school every day. You might have bad days when it is more trouble than it is worth to go out, but don't let your illness turn you into a couch potato.

I'm not particularly athletic. I walk to and from school most days and that's about it. When my lupus flares up, my energy goes way down and I can't even manage that. The nurse in the clinic I go to keeps telling me to get more exercise. I don't see why I should.

I am also a naturally sedentary person, so I understand your reluctance to exercise. There are some reasons why you should, and maybe I can convince you to increase what you are doing.

1. People who exercise regularly have more energy. If you start participating in a physical activity several times a week, you'll find that after a while it acts as a stimulant. You'll feel

the way a coffee drinker feels after the first cup of the day—awake, alert, more alive. (No, I don't think you should just start drinking coffee!)

2. You'll have more muscle strength. Then, when you have a flare-up, maybe you won't be quite as exhausted, because you'll have that extra bit of strength to get up the stairs, or whatever you have to do.

3. You'll feel better about yourself. Despite the fact that you don't enjoy exercise, you probably feel like a bit of a slug when you see other people being more active. As your abilities in your chosen activities improve (and they will, even if you can't participate when you aren't feeling well), your self-esteem will increase. Also, having a chronic condition often leads to a feeling of being out of control. Exercise gives you a level of physical control you may never have experienced.

4. It can help you control your weight when you are on steroids. The more energy your body needs, the more you can take in. You don't have to feel as out of control when you experience those steroid hunger pangs if you know that at least you can control the amount of energy your body uses.

5. It will get the people at the clinic (and probably your parents) off your back about exercising. You won't have to worry before appointments about what excuse to use this time. The clinic staff will have more positive feelings about you. This will make clinic visits less stressful.

Have I convinced you? If so, you need to think about what activity you might be interested in. You could start by increasing your walking. Take a longer route home by walking with a friend who lives a bit out of the way. Go for a walk in the evening with a friend or family member. Get a dog. (Do not, I repeat, do not do this without talking with your parents and then blame it on me! Pets are a big responsibility and getting one must be a family decision.)

Think carefully about what might suit you. You may want the motivation of exercising with other people. You might feel embarrassed to start with a friend, but you could join a class. If you have joint problems, you'll need something low impact and something that will increase flexibility. The climate in your area and your feelings about being outdoors in some seasons will influence whether you want an indoor or an outdoor sport. If you already have a skill (such as swimming or being able to catch a ball), you may want to choose an activity that will build on this.

Talk to your doctor or a physiotherapist at the clinic and find out if there is something you shouldn't do.

Keep your start-up costs down. If you need expensive equipment, rent it until you are sure you like the sport. If you will be going to a gym, find one that has a three-month trial period instead of signing up for five years. Don't push yourself hard every day, but don't make it too easy either. Set up a reasonable schedule.

Give the activity a fair trial, but if you hate it after a few tries, give it up and try something else. Make a rule that you can't quit one thing until you have decided on your replacement activity and have a definite start date.

Your new activities should be recreational, not just good for you, so keep trying things until you find something that you can look forward to doing.

I spend two or three hours a day playing a video game. I do my homework on and off at the same time. I always take my medications on time, so my mother can't say that the game interferes with my

meds. Even still, she complains that I spend too much time playing it. Is there any way that I can get her off my back?

I think you should honestly ask yourself if you are spending too much time gaming. Are you doing worse in school since you started playing? Are you irritable if you can't play? Are you feeling depressed? Do you think about the game when you are at school or with your friends? Are you unwilling to attend special occasions because you wouldn't be playing? Are you having difficulty falling asleep? Have you become overweight? Have you stopped exercising?

If the answer to all these questions is no, then you probably aren't overdoing it. You might want to explain this to your mother, and point out that it doesn't interfere with your meds either.

You probably also watch some TV (or TV shows on your computer), do homework on the computer and go on a social networking site. I do think that we all spend too much time staring at screens. But I also think that you are at an age when you are learning to regulate yourself and how you spend your time. If your mother has noticed changes in your behavior or has other concerns, then I think you should listen to her and set up a schedule where you have some evenings with no games. Otherwise, discuss this with her and point out the ways in which your life is going well, despite the game.

I have what my doctor refers to as "moderate" asthma. (I'm not sure what he means by this— much of the time I'm fine as long as I take my medication, but when I have an attack, there is nothing moderate about it.) I just started high school and my phys ed teacher says I shouldn't

participate. She says the level of activity is higher than in junior high and she could get sued if anything happened to me.

Unfortunately, your gym teacher is quite out of date. Like all teens, you need exercise—for fitness, for fun and to help you feel good about yourself. Just what you don't need is to be singled out as being unable to participate.

It is true that in some people, asthma attacks are brought on by exercise. Cold weather and the stress of competition can also lead to an attack. If you have noticed that you wheeze during or after exercise, when exercising in the cold or when competing, you should talk with your doctor about using medication (oral or inhaled) before these situations.

There is no sport that is absolutely outlawed for asthmatics. You and your doctor can discuss the sports you want to play. There may be days when you are wheezing and can't fully participate, and if you find that one sport always makes you wheeze, you might consider switching to something else. Many teens find that even at times when they are having many attacks they can still swim without experiencing breathing problems. If even swimming brings on an attack, try the backstroke. It is easier to breathe while doing it, and some people find this is the best way for them to swim.

Because it usually takes a few minutes before you start to wheeze, a sport that provides exercise in short bursts (like sprinting, baseball and gymnastics) may be a good choice if you want to be involved in a competitive sport. (Many Olympic athletes have had exercise-induced asthma.)

Ask your doctor to write a letter to the principal of your school (with a copy to your phys ed teacher) stating that you can participate in gym class and outlining the measures you should take if you start to have difficulty breathing. Your gym teacher might feel more comfortable if your parents sign a release stating that she is not responsible if you have breathing problems with normal gym activity. It is your responsibility to let her know if you are having difficulty breathing during class; it is hers to respond appropriately to that information.

By the way, doctors judge the severity of illnesses using a variety of indicators, including how often you get sick, how much medication you need on a regular basis and how bad things are when you get sick.

I am 15 and have pulmonary hypertension (PH). My nurse tells me that I should stay active, but then the doctor tells me all the things I can't do. What's the deal?

Since there are so many activities in the world, it is quite possible that you can be active while not doing the things your doctor says are dangerous. Exercise has been shown to improve stamina in people with PH, so it is a good idea to find ways to get active that are safe. It sounds like your nurse and doctor have very different personalities—the nurse looks at what is positive and the doctor, well, not so much.

There isn't a lot of evidence about exercise and pulmonary hypertension, but we do know that it is important to avoid getting hit in the chest. No football, ice hockey, baseball or boxing. Most specialists would also say no weightlifting or isometric exercises. What does that leave? Swimming, golf and dancing come to mind. But I'm sure you can come up with more.

After a pep talk from a friend, I decided to go swimming with her. I've always loved to swim, but I haven't gone since I got psoriasis. She convinced me that no one would notice my skin when I was in the water, and that we could just ignore anyone in the change room who stared at me. In fact, the change room happened to be empty, so I was feeling like everything was OK. Then, as we were heading to the pool, one of the lifeguards stopped us and said that I couldn't go into the pool because I had a rash. He said I could come back when it was gone. I tried to explain that it wasn't going to go away, but he wouldn't listen. I probably wasn't too clear, because I was crying. My friend called him an insensitive, bureaucratic, self-important, sexist pig (I'm not sure why she put in the sexist part) and we left. It was satisfying to hear her yell at him, and it gave me time to stop crying, but I still can't go to the pool. What can I do?

I am sure that whoever wrote this rule intended it to cover infectious diseases only. I can't think of any other reason why people with rashes might be barred from the pool. The rule may even say "infectious diseases, including rashes and sores," or the person who wrote the rule may have thought that all rashes are catching.

You or one of your parents should call the pool and talk to whoever is in charge. Find out what the exact wording of the rule is. If it just mentions "rash," ask for a justification of this. If the pool is assuming that all rashes are contagious, let the person know this isn't true and that you want the rule changed. Send a letter explaining why the rule must be changed and giving a date by which time you expect some action. Send copies of the letter to the boss of whomever you talked to, the appropriate person at the Public Health Department and anyone else you can think of (maybe the mayor or a city counselor).

If the people at the pool don't get back to you by the date you set, start calling and sending more letters. You may want to threaten to go to the media to tell of the discrimination you are suffering.

Another possibility is that you could ask whoever is in charge of the pool to let you in if you have a letter from your doctor saying you aren't contagious. You will probably have to show it every time there is a lifeguard you don't know.

Hopefully you will be able to get this sorted out quickly and start swimming.

I am incontinent and I have to wear diapers. None of my friends know this, even though they know about some of my other medical problems. I wear loose clothes like sweatpants (fortunately, so do many other guys at our school) and this hides the diaper. Now we have a new coach who says that we can't wear sweatpants in gym class, we have to wear shorts. They can't even be cutoff sweatpants (he says they look sloppy). If I have to wear shorts, my diapers might show when I lean over. Also, they will be bunchy under the shorts and obvious to everyone. What am I going to do?

You, or someone, will need to talk to the coach. I would recommend that you and your father do it together if possible.

The challenge is going to be that this guy sounds very rigid, and to change his mind about this rule, he will have to be flexible.

Talk to him and explain the situation. Make it clear that you expect he will not mention your incontinence to anyone else. He might suggest some options that are not acceptable to you. It is important that you communicate this to him. He might say that he will let you drop gym class or will give you credit for doing something athletic on your own. This may be tempting, but it is a solution that makes *you* the problem, to be dealt with by banishment. He may say that he will make an exception for you and let you wear sweatpants. This would mean that you would be singled out. Your classmates would want to know why you don't have to wear shorts.

The only real solution is for him to relax his rule and let anyone wear sweatpants who wants to. You should give him a chance to come to this idea himself, rather than suggesting it at the beginning. Bring it up only if he has gone through other options and clearly isn't going to think of this one.

If worse comes to worst, he will refuse this as an option and you will have to go to the principal and discuss it with him. If you have a school nurse, see if you can get her on your side and ask her to come to this meeting. You can prepare some arguments why other kids should be able to wear pants (someone may have scars on his legs he doesn't want seen, it is cold in the gym … be creative). Point out that you are not willing to be discriminated against because of your disability, and that you feel it is your right to attend gym classes.

I have CAH (congenital adrenal hyperplasia) and I take steroids every day. I love to run and have been doing well on my school track team. My coach is encouraging me to get even more involved in competitive sports, but if I do I'll be faced with drug testing. I haven't talked to my coach about this, but is there any way for someone on steroids to be allowed to compete?

The steroids that are banned in sports are what are called anabolic steroids and are different from the steroids that are taken to suppress adrenal activity, replace missing steroids in the body or treat a number of conditions. You can take prednisone, prednisalone or cortisol without worrying about competing.

There are a lot of drugs available to teens these days that enhance strength or endurance. Although no one should be using these banned substances, it is particularly important for anyone with a chronic condition to avoid these. There can be interactions with your medications or with your condition. The people who sell these drugs are not exactly the most ethical people around, so you may not always be getting what they say they are selling you.

I have this thing called AIS (androgen insensitivity syndrome), which means that even though I am a girl, I have a Y chromosome, so a blood test would say that I'm a guy, even though I'm not. Does this mean I can't compete at the Olympics?

In the past there were a lot of concerns about men pretending to be women and competing against them. To prove that everyone competing in women's sports were actually women, a number of steps were taken. This sometimes included gynecological exams, competitors having to parade nude in front of a panel of women, blood tests and tests looking at scrapings from the inside of the cheek.

Fortunately, things have changed, at least at the Olympics. It stopped the testing for the Sydney Olympics, knowing that all winners get observed when they give their urine samples and the observer would notice a penis. This trial seems to have gone well, and there has been no indication that they are planning to restart testing.

Now all you have to do is get on the team!

I used to do lots of sports, but then I started having kidney problems. I haven't had much energy and don't participate much. I might be having a transplant soon, and they say I'll have more energy. Will I be able to play sports, or will that damage my kidney?

All the people I've talked to who have had a transplant tell me they do have more energy. Most of them participated in some athletics, and the biggest limiting factor seemed to be their parents' worries. (Many had parents who were happy to see them being active again and had no problems with sports participation.)

Sports that involve fairly violent body contact, like football, boxing, soccer and wrestling, are probably not a good idea. If you can wear a shield (like in hockey), the risks of damage to your kidney are less.

Gymnastics, swimming, baseball, cheerleading, skiing, skating and basketball are all fine.

As it has been quite some time since you were active, you will have to work up to it. Don't expect to be at your old level of energy and ability the day you get home. You are going to have to build up your muscles.

Start with some activities you can do by yourself, like swimming or an exercise program. Make sure you do lots of stretching before you start and again when you are finished.

There are World Transplant Games every two years in a fabulous location. Your transplant team should be able to tell you about where they are, how to get ready and how to fundraise to go. There are probably also national transplant games in your country on the years when there aren't international ones. I know several young people who have medaled!

If you (or anyone) gets mononucleosis, your spleen will get big. With an enlarged spleen, contact sports (or any sport in which you could get bashed in the belly) should be avoided. Instead, stick to things like swimming, cheerleading, badminton, golf and dancing. There are other things that can cause an enlarged spleen, so if your doctor says you have one, ask about sports.

Here are some guidelines for certain conditions not covered in other questions:

Allergies: You may run into problems with outdoor sports in the spring and fall if you have hay fever. Talk to your doctor about medications to prevent your symptoms without making you drowsy.

If you have problems indoors with mold or dust, then mildew in the change room and a poorly cleaned gym could be a problem. You can either get medication or try to get the school to do something about the mildew and dust.

Cardiac Transplant: You will need to work up to activities somewhat gradually. The biggest thing for you to know is that your heart doesn't have a connection to the nerve that used to tell it to speed up. It now knows to get faster because of chemicals that your body makes, but these take longer to have an effect. So you need to have a long warm-up and get your heart rate up before starting an activity. Avoid activities where you have short bursts of energy, as your heart rate won't be able to keep up. Find out what your target heart rate is from your physiotherapist and then check your heart rate to see when you reach the target. Notice how you feel. Are you a bit out of breath but still able to speak? Can you feel your heart beating? Pretty soon you will know when you are in your range by these other things and you won't have to check your heart rate very often.

High Blood Pressure: If this is a mild problem or if it is well controlled, you do not need to restrict your activities. If this is a bigger problem, you should talk with your doctor. She may want to do an exercise test that will look at how high your blood pressure gets when you exert yourself.

Seizures: If you are on medication that controls your seizures well, you do not have to limit your sports. However, if you start to have seizures while participating, you should consider changing sports. If you are having frequent seizures, you should not be involved in body contact sports. No one should swim unsupervised, and this is even more important if you have a seizure disorder. Some doctors feel that "collision sports" in which you are more likely to get a head injury, like boxing, football, hockey and rugby, should be avoided by anyone with epilepsy.

I have cystic fibrosis and I feel too weak to exercise. I don't see how it could be good for me to get all sweaty and short of breath.

There are many things about your disease that you cannot change. It is wise to use your time and your energy (which is pretty limited right now) doing things that can actually improve how you feel. Exercise can improve your endurance (so that you can do more before you get short of breath). Studies have shown that regular exercise actually helps you clear mucus from your lungs. Many people with CF have poor posture, which comes from having to use your shoulder and abdominal muscles to help you breathe. Exercises that strengthen your back muscles and stretch your shoulder and abdominal muscles will improve your posture, helping you to feel more attractive. And, although it can be hard to fit into your schedule, regular exercise can give you time to be with other teens doing normal activities. Scheduling your exercise can help you take control over the rest of your daily schedule.

Consider starting with a Wii or Kinect Sports. You'll be in your home where you can stop and rest easily if you need to. You can gradually increase the level of activity. And your friends will want to do it with you—a big plus.

If you have heart problems or need supplemental oxygen, you should ask your doctor about having an exercise stress test before starting on an exercise program. Even on oxygen, you can do posture exercises and use an exercise bike for short periods of time.

Avoid activities that involve short bursts of great exertion, and go for things that give you a steady level of exercise that raises your heartbeat. Swimming, bicycling and walking are all good for this type of steady exertion. Start with a small amount of exercise at least three times a week and gradually build up.

Set yourself some attainable goals. It might be helpful to talk with a physiotherapist to help plan them. When you have reached them, it is time to set more.

By doing this, you won't be as weak. You may even be able to start seeing yourself as someone who has the strength to take charge of the changeable aspects of your life.

I just got diabetes. My parents think that if I don't do sports, it will be easier to figure out how much insulin I need, and I will be able to be on the same amount every day. I'd like to get back to my old activities. I used to want to be a professional baseball player, but I guess that won't be possible now.

Guess again. There have been professional athletes in every sport you can think of who have had diabetes. This includes baseball players Ty Cobb, Jackie Robinson and Catfish Hunter.

Not only is it OK to be athletic when you're diabetic, it is good for you. It makes your heart stronger and decreases your cholesterol levels. However, you should be in good diabetic control before getting involved in a training program.

Certain sports are harder for your body to adjust to. These include any that involve short, explosive bursts of muscular activity. Baseball can fall into this category, so it is important to warm up well. Try to have a position that requires sustained activity, rather than spending most of your time standing in the outfield.

You will have to pay attention to things like meals and your insulin dosage and timing to make sure you keep your blood sugar in a good range. Both high and low blood sugar can cause problems with strength and coordination. Exercise can mask the symptoms of low blood sugar, so you may not be as aware that you are getting into trouble.

You are, I am sure, already measuring your blood sugar several times a day. Consider checking your blood sugar before and after exercising to get get an idea of the effect of activity. There are apps that will let you connect your glucometer to your cell phone and that will give you a graph of your readings. You can add notes about activity and food. You can take this record to your doctor for help in figuring out what changes you may need to make. He may recommend more frequent insulin injections or a change in their timing.

Keeping your exercise constant throughout the year will allow you to have similar insulin and diet requirements instead of having to change from season to season. You may want to go from baseball to hockey to cross-country running, for instance. If you are less active in the winter, make sure you monitor your blood sugar closely in the spring when you start to get involved in sports again, or you could end up with a dangerously low blood sugar.

You may absorb insulin more quickly if you are exercising the part of your body that you injected it into. Inject in your thighs at times when you aren't going to be active, and into your belly before games and practices. If you use your arm, use the one you don't throw with.

It is important to get plenty to eat after exercising, or your blood sugar could drop while you are asleep and unable to notice. Check your blood sugar before going to bed if you think you didn't eat enough. Having a snack before exercising can also help keep your blood sugar at a more even level. Have some chocolates or a sweet drink available, and if you are going to be involved in a longer activity, like cross-country running or skiing, eat or drink something high in sugar while you are exercising.

Don't drink alcohol when you are in training. It can lower your blood sugar.

Exercising in the morning tends to lower your blood sugar for the rest of the day. This may mean you will need less insulin or that you can eat a bit more.

Your coach should know that you are diabetic and what this means. Your doctor or someone else at the clinic where you go may be able to talk to your coach about improving your glucose levels during training and games.

Your coach may recommend that your teammates practice carbohydrate loading for three days before a big game. This is not a good idea for you.

If you develop eye problems (proliferative retinopathy) in the future, then you will have to stop most sports activities. Increases in your blood pressure while exercising or getting bashed around could cause a hemorrhage in your eye. The better your diabetic control, the less likely you are to develop this problem, although it isn't totally protective.

The more you understand about where energy comes from during exercise and how your muscles use it, the better you will be able to participate in managing your exercise/insulin/diet routine.

Your parents are right that you will need to pay extra attention to your blood sugar control as an athlete. This extra effort is worth the payoff—getting to participate in activities, seeing yourself as a person whose activities aren't limited by diabetes, getting to eat more and better overall health.

Because of my illness I weigh less than most guys my age, and I'm shorter. I like to wrestle and I'm pretty good at it. When the team practices at school, I wrestle people my own age and get a good workout. When we wrestle at other schools or in tournaments, I end up wrestling much younger and inexperienced kids, because we're classified by weight. It's not much fun for me and I don't think it is fair to them. Is there anything I can do about this?

This is an unfortunate situation that you are not going to be able to change. Categories for wrestling matches are defined by weight to try to match up competitors. They don't take into account people who are either at a disadvantage because they are big but inexperienced or people who are smaller and more experienced. You are not going to get the sport changed because you and a few other people have an unfair advantage.

I don't think you should give up wrestling because of this. You get to wrestle with people you are matched with in skill at practices. If you go on to wrestle after you finish high school, you will be competing against other adults, and the people in your weight category will be around your age or older. You are gaining valuable experience wrestling with your larger teammates, and you are helping the younger people you compete against develop their skills.

Don't assume that you always have the advantage or you'll get clobbered one of these days. You are not the only smaller-than-average guy who wrestles.

I am being encouraged (that is, pushed) to go on an Outward Bound-type trip. You know, live off the land, jump off mountains, that kind of thing. The whole idea scares me. Why should I go?

The whole idea scares me too, but I think that is the point. You go and do something that is scary and learn that you are capable of facing and overcoming the things that you feared.

Going on a trip like this will help you feel more in control of your body and your life. It will help you feel better about yourself. There is an old saying, "Nothing succeeds like success." As you accomplish things you thought you were incapable of, you will feel better and better about yourself.

On an adventure like this, your body becomes a tool you use to surmount difficulties, rather than something you are fighting against.

You get away from your family for a week or two, and get to be with people your own age. You will be with people who don't see you as being excessively limited by your condition. You will discover that you have more in common with other teens and are less different than you thought.

After the program, you will probably be more willing to take physical risks, and your parents are more likely to see you as being capable of these things. Chances are you will get more involved in other recreational activities.

If there are any special instructions about your condition (like if you get sick or have a flare), print them out and laminate them (you can often find a laminator at bus stations or drug stores). The leaders must be informed about your condition and anything that needs to be changed to accommodate your condition. Make sure you take a waterproof container for your medications, and give a second set to one of the leaders.

Everybody I have talked with who has gone on a program like this has enjoyed it immensely, even those who initially didn't want to go.

I play wheelchair basketball and I keep getting blisters on my hands, then I can't play until they heal. Is there anything I can do about this?

Sports injuries are fairly common in wheelchair basketball, road racing and track. One of the most common injuries is blistering of the hands.

Blisters are caused by friction on your skin; you'll often feel some discomfort before you get a blister.

You can prevent blisters in a few ways. One is to gradually toughen the skin on your hands. If you play basketball once a week and do little in between, start doing daily training. After a good warm-up (stretching your arms, neck and back), wheel quickly around a track. When your hands start to hurt, stop right away, even if it has only been a couple of minutes. Every day you should be able to go a bit longer, and eventually you will build up calluses on your hands; the calluses will protect the skin on your hands.

You can also protect your hands during games by wearing gloves. Leather driving gloves are a good choice, as are cycling gloves. They have holes in them, so your hands won't stay as sweaty, and they fit closely, so your hands won't slip.

Some people tape the areas where they tend to get blisters.

Many sports injuries can be prevented with careful training, good warm-up and cool-down exercises, and protective clothing.

I want to learn how to drive, but my parents think I shouldn't. They say they are happy to take me anywhere, but that isn't the point. This is something I want to be able to do for myself. Since I am old enough to get my learner's permit, shouldn't they let me get it?

Your parents may have a variety of reasons for not wanting you to learn to drive. They may be worried about your chances of succeeding. They may not be aware that people with a wide range of illnesses and disabilities have learned to drive. If they feel you can't succeed, they may worry it would be bad for your self-esteem. An evaluation of your ability to drive would be helpful in convincing them.

It is probably hard for your parents to let go and allow you to be independent. They may have got into the habit of taking care of you, and the degree of independence involved with driving may be threatening to them. This can be particularly true if you are the oldest in your family (it is hard to let the first kid learn to drive) or the youngest (once you can drive, they don't have a "baby of the family" anymore).

Your parents may have noticed some things about you that make them worry about your ability to drive. Driving has as much to do with decision making as it does with mechanics. They may have concerns about your decision-making skills. You can work on showing them that you are capable of taking responsibility and deciding things if you think this is their concern.

If you have a hard time controlling your temper, your parents may feel it isn't a good idea for you to drive. A person who is angry and behind the wheel of a car is dangerous. People can be badly hurt or killed as a result of an angry driver. If anger control is a problem of yours, you could ask the social worker at the clinic you go to to recommend a course in anger management. Once you know how to deal with your anger, you will be a safer driver.

Are you sure you are ready to drive? Sixteen is not the magic age for everyone. I learned to drive when I was 20. I waited until I could afford a car. I don't think it had any lasting effect on me to have waited. If your interests lie in the area of people and not math and physics, learning to drive may be more difficult.

You need your parents' support to learn to drive. They are the ones who will go out with you so that you can practice, and you may need them to get you to your lessons. Try to figure out why your parents are worrying about this. If it is something about your behavior that you think is making them uneasy, try to start the process of changing. If you feel that they are scared to let you become more independent, you may have to confront them about this. Either way, you can start to prepare to learn how to drive. The reply to the next question gives some tips.

I am on a waiting list for a driver's ed course and will be starting in four months. I have cerebral palsy but my doctor says I should be OK to drive. Is there anything I can do to get ready for it?

Good question. It is very wise to prepare to learn to drive. As I have pointed out in the preceding reply, there is more to driving than mechanics, and you can work on increasing your skills in various areas.

You need to work on your ability to make independent decisions. You may want to increase your responsibilities around the house and take on some chores that involve making decisions, like making shopping lists or doing the shopping. See if your parents will let you have a party for which you do all the planning.

Try to improve your coordination if you can. Any sports involvement will help with this, whether it's team or individual. Playing computer games, especially ones that you haven't already mastered, may help. If you haven't learned to type, this could be a good time.

Ask your guidance counselor if there is anything in your school record about your having a "visual-spatial" problem. This is common in people with cerebral palsy and spina bifida. If you do, you may have problems judging how far away things are and how fast you and other cars are traveling. If you do have problems in this area, talk to an occupational therapist to see if there are some exercises you can do to improve your ability to judge distances and speeds.

Read the driver's handbook for your province or state. Keep rereading it until you can remember everything in it. Have a friend quiz you (and return the favor if he or she is learning to drive). Many driver's handbooks are available in an easy-to-read format, with large type, lots of pictures and understandable language. (The one in Ontario is called *The Ontario Driver's Manual Adapted for Adult New Readers.*)

Practice something called "commentary passengering." Sit in the front seat and pretend you are the driver. Talk to whoever is driving about what you would be noticing if you were driving (you need to discuss this in advance, so it's clear you aren't telling him or her how to drive). You'll be mentioning what other cars are doing, pedestrians, stop signs, yellow and red lights, and stray animals. You will be trying not to notice billboards, stores, friends or other non-essentials. Try to guess whether your car or others have time to make left-hand turns or go through a light without speeding up.

If you are shorter than average, build up your seat with cushions so that you are high enough to see over the dashboard.

If you use crutches, you may be used to keeping your eyes lowered so you're looking at the ground while walking. Train yourself to keep your eyes looking ahead, not down at the sidewalk. When driving, you have to be able to look ahead, and not just be staring at the road right in front of you.

Make up games where you guess how far things are, or how big they are. Start with distances in your house, like guessing how big a room is. Check your guess by measuring it. When in the car, ask your parent to say "start" when the odometer says that a new kilometer (or mile) has started. The you say when you think a certain distance has passed.

If you feel fairly prepared, you may be able to take the theory part of a driver's course at your school. This will all be repeated when you take the other course, but it can be helpful to hear things more than once.

To be able to drive well, you must be mature and assertive (not aggressive). There is no specific way to learn maturity. It comes from having a variety of life experiences, from dealing with difficult issues, and from developing a worldview that is broader than just how things affect you.

My guidance counselor at school has been encouraging me to learn how to drive. I'm sure I could never afford a special car, so why bother?

It is often useful to learn a new skill, even if you can't afford to use it right away. If you could get access to a car you could drive, it would open up many possibilities in your life. You may have more educational choices, a larger choice of jobs, better job security (if you have to rely on other people to get you to work, there is a higher chance of being late) and an improved social life. Although many people get along fine without driving, it can be quite useful.

Have you checked into the price of vehicle modifications? If you are assuming that it will be expensive, you may be in for a pleasant surprise. Modifications can probably be done to your parents' car (they can still drive it), so unless you want exclusive use of the car, the only costs will be the modifications, insurance and driver's education.

For many people, the only modifications that need to be made are hand controls, which are around $500 - $700. If all you need is a left-foot gas pedal; this is usually under $400. An extended pedal (which you may need if you are short) is more costly, $1,000 or more.

Many North American car makers give a rebate of $500 to $1,000 for modifications. Check into this if you are buying a car. You may be able to get a rebate from the government for the sales tax you pay on this work.

In some areas, there are associations (like Easter Seals) that will help pay for driver education.

You need to have an evaluation to see what you would need. There are centers throughout North America that perform these evaluations—your rehab doctor can help you connect with the nearest one. Some people do need expensive modifications, but many need only minor changes.

I use a wheelchair. If I learn how to drive, will I have to get one of those special vans?

Many people with wheelchairs drive regular cars. Four-door cars often have front doors that don't open wide enough, so a two-door car is your best bet. You will need to shop around for a car that you can get in and out of and get your wheelchair in behind you.

If you can afford it, a van has the advantages of wide doors and plenty of space to put stuff. Minivans are often lower to the ground than full-sized vans.

My sister says I shouldn't drive because I don't see so well. I don't want to do anything dangerous, but I would love to be able to drive a car.

Check with your local authorities; the common rule is that your visual acuity in your best eye, while wearing your glasses or contacts, is at least 20/40, and that you only have to have vision in one eye. You can go to your eye doctor and get this checked. If your eyesight isn't this good, talk to your doctor and see if there is any way to further improve your vision.

In addition to having to be able to see fairly well with one eye, you also need 120° of peripheral vision. This is how far you can see to the side when you are looking straight ahead. Your eye doctor can check your peripheral vision for you.

Your eyes also have to be able to work well together and move well.

I hope you will be able to qualify for a driving test. If you can't, remember that alternative ways of getting around are helpful for the environment. Your vision doesn't need to be as good to bike, and, needless to say, there is no sight requirement for riding the bus, train or streetcar.

I take medication and I worry that it will interfere with my ability to drive. How can I find out more about this?

If your medication makes you feel sleepy, or if you have noticed problems in coordination with it, you might not be able to drive. Although many drugs have drowsiness as a side effect, it is usually something that goes away after you have been using the drug for a couple of weeks.

If your medications are changed or your dosage is increased (or if your glasses' prescription is changed), it is a good idea to wait two to three weeks to make sure that you have adjusted to the change.

Your doctor should be able to tell you if your medication is a problem.

No one should drink and drive, but this is especially important if you are on medication or if you have had a head injury. If you drink alcohol, you may be impaired as a driver before you reach the legal limit.

I have epilepsy and my family doctor says this means I will never be able to drive. To me, this is a terrible thought. I feel like I'll be stuck living in places with good public transportation for the rest of my life, and I have always wanted to live in the country.

There are restrictions for drivers with seizure disorders everywhere in North America. Every province and state has its own rules. In many places, you can start driving if you have gone a year without a seizure. In others, the wait is longer.

It is important that you abide by this. It may be tempting to lie about seizures, maybe even to try to hide them from your family and your doctor. There are real dangers involved in having a seizure while driving. Even if you think you have plenty of warning, you cannot count on this. Too much is at stake.

You may have to make some big decisions. There may be a medication with side effects that drive you crazy but that medication keeps you free of seizures. If driving weren't an issue, you might be willing to have the occasional seizure and be on a medication that is easier to tolerate. To be able to drive, you may opt to take the drug with more side effects.

I am deaf and I am in a "regular" school. All my friends are learning to drive. I've always thought that I couldn't drive, but I'd like to be able to.

There are many good drivers who are deaf or hearing impaired. You may have an advantage over other teens, as you will not be distracted by noises. It is important for all drivers to see what is going on around them and to really pay attention. You have a lifetime of experience in doing this.

Are there times when a deaf driver is at a disadvantage? People often honk at drivers who are driving dangerously or when they are in danger. This honking can alert a driver to the danger. A deaf driver would not hear this warning. The solution, of course, is to not drive dangerously—don't back up if you can't see behind you, check your mirrors frequently and assume that pedestrians won't use common sense.

Sirens are important warnings that emergency vehicles are on the way. Many people who are deaf can hear sirens, as they are loud and the sound moves through many frequencies. Even if you can't hear them, these vehicles also have flashing lights, so if you are paying attention to what is going on ahead of and behind you, and you are careful at intersections, you should be fine.

8 Transitions

AS WE GO THROUGH LIFE, things change constantly. Some of the changes are small, some are major. Some of these transitions happen only to people with illnesses (like going from being healthy to having some kind of diagnosis), and some are things that happen to almost everybody, like going to a new school, moving to a different city or getting a job. These transitions may be more significant, or harder to deal with, if you are also coping with a chronic condition. This last chapter looks at some of the issues related to change and how to deal with it. Sometimes, when you live with an illness or disability, you get used to changes being bad. It often seems that changes in one's condition are changes for the worse, and it becomes easy to assume that life changes will also be negative. While major changes can be hard, they can often be positive, a sign of growth and learning. Try not to make too many negative assumptions about the changes that come your way.

I got diabetes when I was 12 and went to the clinic at a children's hospital. I really felt ready to get out of there last year when I turned 18. I only went once to the endocrinologist they sent me to. I really didn't feel comfortable with him, and I didn't get the feeling that he saw me as a person. I'm away at college and my parents keep bugging me to get a new doctor. I know I should, but I don't know how to find someone I like. Can you help me?

It can be hard to find a new doctor, especially as doctors who treat adults tend to have a different style from those treating younger patients. It is important to get a doctor, and when you find someone you like, there will be some advantages to the adult model of care.

Call the college health center to see if it has a list of family doctors and endocrinologists in your area who are interested in diabetes. Put up a sign at the health center or on bulletin boards in highly trafficked areas asking other diabetic students to get in touch with you, and when they do, ask who their doctor is.

Make a list of what is important to you about a doctor's office. These may be things such as evening hours and having someone on call for the practice instead of just a tape telling you to go to a hospital's emergency department. Methods of payment are also important. When you've completed this list, call the offices of the doctors whose names you have collected and ask these questions. Cross off the doctors who can't meet these expectations.

Now make another list. What is important to you in a doctor? Someone who will treat you in a humane manner? Someone who is up on the latest research? Someone who can explain things well? Someone who sees you as a partner in your care? Make appointments with the remaining doctors on your list. Let the office staff know you want to just talk with the doctor. When you go for the appointment, ask the doctor questions about her philosophy of treatment. Get a feel for what the person is like. You may not have to go through your whole list of doctors. If you find someone you feel comfortable with, you can stop your search (just remember to cancel your other appointments).

This sounds like a daunting task, but you are looking for someone you can stick with for quite some time. There may be only two or three doctors on your final list. The whole process probably won't take any longer than writing a research paper.

The nurse at my clinic has been going on about "getting ready to move to adult care." I don't really see what the big deal is. I mean, it's a hospital, it will have the same uncomfortable beds, terrible food and expensive parking. It's not going to be that different.

There are many similarities between pediatric and adult care settings. Some people even continue to get their care in the same building, just moving from the children's clinic and ward to the adult ones. Many young people look forward to getting away from the cartoon characters on the walls, the Disney videos and the tiny chairs.

There are also real differences between the two. They aren't usually obvious—it's like moving to a country where everyone speaks the same language. Everything looks the same, people sound the same, but after a while you realize that there is a different culture. One of the main differences between the two is that pediatric care is family-centered, with health care providers talking with parents, including them in planning and really seeing the whole family as the patient. Adult care tends to be more patient-centered. It's not that the health care providers won't talk with family members, but their focus is on you. They will expect you to be in charge of your medications and your health and to be making your own decisions about your care.

Adult centers tend to have a lot more patients and most of them will be older, even elderly.

You will be expected to entertain yourself—no child life workers or teen lounge. You will probably have to rent a TV if you want one.

To succeed in the adult system, you will need to be able to talk with health care providers, and to be prepared with your questions or concerns when you go to appointments. You will have to speak up for yourself. You will learn to find resources outside the hospital, as adult hospitals tend to have fewer social workers and psychologists than children's hospitals.

On the other hand, you will be in a place where you are treated like an adult. Your providers will assume that, as an adult, you are either in, or may be looking for, a relationship. They won't be shocked to find out that you have sex. Expect that they will welcome you (and your family) into their care, treat you with respect and not have any tiny chairs in the waiting room.

I have been in hospital many times and have had surgery and all kinds of procedures. My hospital chart is into its third volume! Now I'm going to be moving on to another doctor. How am I going to answer her questions about what I've had done? I'm not even sure how many procedures I've had.

It is important that you be able to tell your new health care workers what has happened to you. You need to take a two-pronged approach to this. One is for you to be able to tell the major stuff to whoever needs to know it. The second is to have a detailed summary of your care.

For you to be able to tell your story, you need to be able to put the important parts into a very short format. I call this the three-sentence summary. You will state the name of your diagnosis, when you got sick, major complications and what meds you are on now. You probably know all this, but put it all together and practice saying it. You can then back this up with more detailed information on a MyHealth Passport. Go to the website at www.sickkids.ca/myhealthpassport, pick the template for your condition and then fill in the info. You can then print it, cut it out and fold it into a wallet-sized card. You can also e-mail it to yourself.

But neither the three-sentence summary nor the MyHealth Passport will have the level of detail that should be communicated to your new doctor and hospital. Ask your current doctor to write a summary of all operations, procedures and important lab work you've had done. Let her know that you want a copy for yourself. The next time you see her, ask her if she's done it yet. It is a very boring task to sift through all that information, and doctors have a tendency to put off doing it. If she says she'll send it directly to the other doctor and doesn't want to give a copy to you, explain that you feel it is important you have this information yourself. You may not stay with this new doctor, and even if you do, it might be important to you at some point to know exactly what has happened to you. When you get it, make a few copies. If your parents have a safety deposit box, you might ask them to put one in there. Wherever you keep them, they shouldn't all be in the same place.

If your doctor won't give you a copy, you can go to the medical records department at the hospital and find out what your options are. Although most hospitals will give you a copy of your chart, you usually have to pay for it. You end up paying for pages and pages of irrelevant charting, and it can get expensive. It may be hard for you to find the important information buried in all that paper. Hospitals have varying policies about who gives consent to release your chart, and even if you are over 16 you may have to get your parents' consent. Psychiatric records will probably not be released without consent of the person who wrote the notes. Some hospitals will provide a short summary listing operations and procedures and their dates. They might charge for this, but it will be cheaper than getting the whole chart, and they do the work of identifying what is important. Again, make copies.

My parents just told me that we are moving to a much smaller city in a month. They said that it will be a much better environment, safer, with clean air and lots of space. It sounds awfully dull, and my parents think that is why I don't want to move. I always thought that the people in small towns were like the ones in big cities, just not so many of them. When my parents were house hunting, I went to my new school—what a difference from where I go now. I had never noticed, but the school I go to has a wide variety of people. The kids are from all over the world. There is an integrated program for kids who are developmentally handicapped. There are other kids who have various difficulties. Half the school seems to use puffers before gym so they won't wheeze. Dullsville Collegiate isn't like this. I didn't hear any languages besides English being spoken, and almost everyone was white. The friends I have now don't see my illness as being important, but if these kids have never known anyone who is different from them, will they want to be friends with me? Also, there's no children's hospital, and if I have to go on dialysis it will be with a bunch of adults. We visited the hospital and they don't have any teens on dialysis there. I know I can't stop the move, but is there anything I can do to make things better?

Moving is always hard, especially at your age. It can be difficult to make new friends, and most people find that it takes at least a year to adjust to a new situation.

There are things you can do to make the move easier. You have to realize that about 8% of North American kids have a chronic condition, so there will be kids at your school who are "different" in this way. I'm sure you'll see as many puffers before gym class in Dullsville as you do now.

Almost every disease that kids can get has an organization to go with it. Go on the Kidney Foundation website and see if there is a Dullsville chapter. If there is, call the contact person and find out if there are any people around your age in the group and see if you can meet them. If they don't have anyone your age, find out from those in the social work department at your hospital if they know of any groups for kids with chronic conditions. If there aren't any, ask them to start one. See if there is a Facebook or other social networking site with a group for your condition and then try to find someone there from the Dullsville area.

There is nothing you can do about the lack of ethnic diversity in Dullsville, but diversity isn't always visible. Your school will have kids from different socioeconomic backgrounds and family structures. People will have different interests. You have to take diversity where you find it (and go to the city for visits when things seem too white). If there is more than one high school, one might have more obvious diversity than the other. Find out as much as you can about the schools before choosing one.

My friends are all getting ready to go to university, community colleges, the armed forces, or to travel when we graduate from high school in a few months. I am going to stay home, because I need help for my treatments, and I get panicky at the idea of not having my parents around in an emergency. I'd like to go to university, but I didn't apply because I didn't want to waste my parents' money on something I might not be able to use. At the same time, I feel like a baby, staying home and being taken care of.

You've brought up a number of issues. You seem to be assuming that all your friends are going to leave home. Considering the current state of the economy, I'm sure that at least some of them will stay at home while attending school. It is becoming much more common for young people to stay at home until they finish their education.

You seem to think there is something wrong with not being ready to move out. It can be hard to see friends taking wing before you do, but we all move at our own speed.

Perhaps you are afraid that you will never move out. If you want to be more independent but are worried that you can't be, this is a good time to think this through, maybe with the help of an occupational therapist. She can help you figure out the skills you need in order to be out on your own. Maybe you can do your own treatments, or there may be public funding available to pay for someone to help. You will need to consider whether you want to live on your own or with roommates. Maybe you can do this in stages. Is there part of your house that you can turn into a bachelor apartment? Your parents would still be close if you needed them, but you would have some independence. If there are things that are really bugging you, such as a curfew you feel you have outgrown, maybe your parents would be willing to relax or let go of these rules.

University is not typically a trade school. You go to learn, and many people do not learn things they can "use" in any practical sense. In addition, how do you know that you won't be able to? If the costs of your care have been so high that your parents can't afford to send you, you might be able to get a scholarship. If they can afford to send you to university, you should talk to them about going. They may not agree that you would be wasting their money.

If you think it would be a waste of money because you have been told that you are likely to die in the next few years, it is important for you to realize that you can go to university because you would enjoy it now, and that there doesn't have to be a future in it. Besides, what if you live for 20 years? You wouldn't want to spend all that time doing nothing just in case you die. If you don't live to a ripe old age, your parents will have the comfort of knowing that you achieved something that was important to you and that they helped, and you will have the satisfaction of undertaking something important to you.

Don't treat your life as if it is over. It is OK to be scared about moving out, and it is OK to stay at home, if that is what you decide will suit you best. But if you plan your days with the assumption that you are going to live, then each one of them will be fuller and more satisfying.

I have decided to turn my life around. I feel that I have spent the past two years whining "Poor me, poor me." What is the best way for me to fight what my body is doing to me? Everyone gives me advice—meditation, vegetarianism, eat more meat, live on yogurt and grapefruit, do karate and on and on. How do I know what is best?

It is terrific that you have decided to change your life. It is easy to get self-involved and to spend much of your time feeling sorry for yourself, but as you have discovered, it gets boring, and it probably doesn't help you get any better.

Each of us finds our own ways of helping ourselves. You may want to try out various things, but don't do anything that seems unappealing just because someone heard about someone else with exactly the same condition you have who got better after they sent their life savings to someone they heard on TV.

There is something you need to do that is more basic than any of the suggestions your friends have made. You need to change your attitude about yourself.

Your body is you—not all of you, I know, but it isn't some evil thing that has moved in next door and is making you miserable. Something has caused your condition. Maybe you know what it is, maybe not. But you have to help your body, not fight it. If you decide to start jogging, it has to be because you want to make yourself stronger, not because you want to beat down your body.

As long as your body is the enemy, who is your friend? Take care of yourself, be nice to yourself, listen to what your body has to say to you. This doesn't mean that you have to make your condition into your career. There are many important things about you, and about life, and if all you let yourself be is "disabled" or "sick," then you will miss out on many other things. But don't find the time for these things by ignoring your body or hating it.

If you can't see your body as part of yourself, at least learn to view it as a fellow traveler, a companion through this journey. If you act friendly to it, you are more likely to have a comfortable trip.

I have always tried to make it clear to my relatives and friends that if I need help, I will ask for it. I don't take this to stupid extremes. If someone goes through a door ahead of me, I don't expect them to slam it in my face, and I always hold the door if I am the first through it. But I don't expect to be waited on, and I don't want my disability to be the deciding factor in decisions. The people I know well have gone along with this, and I think it makes their lives, as well as mine, easier, because they don't have to second-guess me. My problem is the people who don't know me. As I move out into the world more and more (I will be living in a different city next year), I come into contact with strangers

more. Yesterday, someone grabbed my arm as I was crossing the street and pulled me across. I almost hit her with my cane. I'm sure she meant well, and I don't want to be rude to anyone, but how can I stop people from doing things like this?

When people ask you if you need a hand, I think they are trying to be helpful and are also recognizing that you are a human being who can make decisions about your needs. When people start doing things "for" you, I think they are fulfilling some need of their own. You are under no obligation to allow them to push you around just because it makes them feel good.

You can start by saying, "Thank you, I don't need any help," while pulling your arm away. If they persist, try "Let go of me" in a firm voice. If they still don't let go, and you still don't want to be rude, say, "You are assaulting me. Let go or I will scream."

If the person doesn't touch you but insists on helping, just keep explaining that you don't need help. You do not have to justify yourself and you can leave, even if the person is in the middle of a sentence.

Some people are always doing things "for" other people without considering their needs. If you are being bugged by someone who is like this at work or school, you may want to get together with other people who are being "helped" by this person. Try to work out a strategy. Maybe you can all find errands for him that take him to the other end of the building.

My sister died last year. It was a terrible time for all of us, but I am getting on with my life. I have the same condition as she did, so that has made it harder. My mother doesn't seem to be willing to start doing any of the things we used to. I know I'm a teen and supposed to be independent, but I like

going on family picnics, shopping with my mother and other stuff. Now she just mopes around. From the way she treats me, I am starting to wonder if she wishes that I had died instead of Jane.

Your mother sounds very depressed. This is not surprising, but it is taking its toll on your family.

Your mother is not wishing that you had died, but I'm sure she's wishing that your sister hadn't. Probably a part of her always hoped that a cure would be found, or that both her children would defy all odds and have a normal life span. In addition to being depressed about Jane's death, your mother may be worrying that she will lose you too. She may be grieving about this, which would add to her depression.

When people are depressed, they don't just feel sad. They may not want to eat, and have difficulty sleeping, or sleep more than they used to. They move through life surrounded by a thick fog that prevents them from enjoying things. It can be almost impossible for them to plan to go out on a family outing.

It would help your mother if she got some therapy or joined a group for parents who have lost a child. If she is unwilling or unable to do this, you can see a counselor who can help you find ways to cope with what things are like in your family right now. Your doctor can help you find someone to talk with.

If you live with other family members, you may want to initiate some activities like picnics. Invite your mother to attend, but go even if she says no. Hopefully she'll be able to join you at some point and you'll have helped hold the rest of your family together. If you don't live with other family members, try to firm up your ties with relations you don't live with.

My parents never talk about death. They don't even say the word. JoJo, my cat, died last week and they

haven't mentioned his name since. They took him away to the vet and had him "put down" and I never saw him again. His food bowls and litter seemed to just disappear. From talking with the other kids in the waiting room at the clinic, I've figured out that I am unlikely to live past my twenties. This really scares me, and I'd like to talk about it with someone, but my parents wouldn't be able to cope. I never see my doctor alone. What can I do?

When I was in nursing school I had a five-year-old patient who had leukemia. He was dying, and his parents said that no one was to talk with him about it. They said he was too young to understand and that he wouldn't be able to cope. One day he said to his nurse, "I'm going to die. Don't tell my parents. It would upset them too much." The parents thought he needed to be protected, and their silence convinced him that they needed to be protected.

It may be that your parents really can't cope with the idea of death, and that if you bring it up they'll run out of the room crying, but I think it is more likely that they are tougher than that. They may unconsciously feel that if they never talk about death it won't happen, but of course, it happens to all of us.

Not only are you scared, your parents are too. When we have children we assume that they will outlive us, and it is a terrifying thing for parents to face when this is not how things turn out.

I think there are probably three things you need to do. You need to get some information. You need to talk with someone about how you are feeling. You need to help your parents move beyond their silence.

The information part is important. What you have picked up in the waiting room may not be accurate. Will you die from this illness? When is it likely to happen? Will it all happen very quickly, or will you have some warning that things are getting worse? Will you be in pain? Will you have to be in the hospital or can you be at home? I'm sure you can think of many other questions.

Although your doctor will not be able to tell you when you will die, she will be able to answer many of your questions. You will have to decide whether to ask to speak with her alone or whether you should ask in front of your mother or father. My feeling is that the sense of secrecy in your family about death is not healthy and that you should bring it up in front of them. After you get some facts, you can tell your doctor that you would like to be able to talk with someone about how you are feeling. As you go through this, you will find yourself mentioning death at home occasionally. Once the ice is broken, your parents should be able to open up and talk more. If they don't, you may want to ask them to come with you to an appointment with your counselor. Eventually, they may even be able to talk with you about JoJo.

I am dying. Not in the next few days or anything, but soon. The whole thing really pisses me off, it seems so unfair, but I've been trying not to take this out on my parents. I know that they, and my friends and relatives, are feeling as overwhelmed by this as I am. I want you to settle an argument we are having: I don't want to have a funeral. I feel that it will be hard for all these people to get together who are feeling so bad, and I want to spare them the pain. What do you think?

I think you aren't going to like my answer. To start with, you aren't going to have a funeral, your parents are. You won't be there. Now, you are trying to think of their feelings, but before we talk about that, let's talk about your feelings. Do you really hope your friends and family won't be upset when you die? The only way to make this happen would be to have totally cut yourself off from them, to have lived a life that would make them feel happy that you died. Presumably they are going to be upset because you have been a loving, contributing member of your family and your community.

Now, let's talk about their feelings. These friends are going to be grieving intensely when you die. They need to be able to express that grief, to talk about you and what you meant to them. It will help your friends to be able to show their support for your family. In all cultures, there are rituals that ease us through the important transitions of life. They are observed around the time of birth, becoming an adult, graduating from school, settling down with someone and when we die. Your community will have rituals that will help you in this process—taking care of your family's needs so that they can be with you instead of wasting time cooking, visiting you and maybe bringing flowers or music. The rituals that happen after you die are just as important to your family. By asking them to not have a funeral, you are asking them to not have this one bit of comfort.

You might want to consider planning your funeral with your parents or some close friends. The process might help you deal with some of the overwhelming feelings you are having. Dying is, as I am sure you have already discovered, a process, not something that happens in an instant. By planning the funeral, you take control over a part of this process, and it may lead you to discover other ways to be actively involved, rather than having dying be something that is being done to you.

I was diagnosed with a serious illness a few months ago. Everyone seems to think I'm coping pretty well because I go to all my appointments

and take my medications. But I'm not coping well at all. The other teens I've met at the clinic seem to accept that this illness is a part of them and are just getting on with things. I don't mean that they don't complain about some of the doctors and nurses, or that they always do what they are supposed to, but they seem comfortable with seeing themselves as having a disease. I feel like I am a healthy, strong person and I can't accept that this isn't true anymore.

As you grow up you develop an image of who you are. This is molded by your personality, the way you are viewed within your family, your dreams, your strengths and your weaknesses. People who are diagnosed with an illness or disability at a young age incorporate this into their self-image. (Whether this is a positive or a negative depends on the other factors.) When something about ourselves changes, it takes our self-image a while to catch up, and the process can be painful. This is what you are going through.

One of the things that makes this difficult is that it can be hard to believe that anything we thought we knew about ourselves is no longer. So, you used to feel healthy, now you don't. Maybe you are also wondering if you really have some of the other positives that you took for granted before.

You are essentially the same person you always have been. The experiences you have because of your illness will change how you continue to develop as a person, but you are building on what you had before.

Are you going too far in this adjustment? You seem to be assuming that you are now weak and ill, as opposed to strong and healthy. Does this mean you've been given no hope of feeling better? Tom Koch, whom I met on Ability Online, said,

"It is unfair. It's a raw deal. It means life will never be the same. But will you die tomorrow? If the answer is 'No, certainly not!' I say good, because tomorrow at least will be interesting."

You have to do what you can to figure out in what ways life has not changed. You need to know what your capabilities are. This book is full of suggestions about the things in your life that can be normal. Find out what you're able to do in sports and other activities that are important to you.

Give yourself time. It takes most teens a year to adjust to moving to a new home and school. You are facing a bigger adjustment, so don't expect to be at the place where the teens at the clinic are. They have had longer to adjust. As new people are diagnosed, you will see how far you have come, as you compare how you feel then to how they are doing.

Am I going to be able to find my own ways of being independent and actually turn into a mature person with some control over my life?

Yes.

Will it ever be easy?

Not often, but it will get easier.

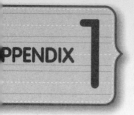

Stuff to Know About Medications

By Nadya Nalli and Miriam Kaufman

Always check with your doctor or pharmacist if you think a medication might be causing a side effect, as we couldn't list every medication that has ever had a side effect.

A	Medications That Can Cause Acne	
ACTH (corticotrophin)	Ethambutol	Phenytoin
Actinomycin D	Ethionamide	Potassium Iodide
Anabolic steroids	Granulocyte colony	Prednisone
(e.g., testosterone,	stimulating factor	Quinidine
nandrolone)	(G-CSF)	Quinine
Androgens	Infliximab	Rifampin
Atorvastatin	Isoniazid (INH)	Sirolimus
Bromides	Lamotrigine	Topiramate
Cyclosporine	Lithium	Trimethadione
Danazol	Phenobarbital	Valganciclovir

B	Medications That Can Cause Hairiness (to Varying Degrees)	
Acetazolamide	Diazoxide	Prednisone
Acyclovir	Diltiazem	Prochloperazine
Amlodipine	Erythropoietin	Progesterone
Anabolic steroids	Methoxsalen	Sirolimus
(e.g., testosterone,	Metoclopramide	Thioridazine
nandrolone)	Minoxidil	Tretinoin
Androgens	Nimodipine	(retinoic acid)
Cyclosporine	Oral contraceptives	Valproic acid
Danazol	Penicillamine	Verapamil
Dexamethasone	Phenytoin	Zidovudine

C | Medications That Can Cause Decreased Sexual Desire

Acetazolamide	Doxepin	Metoclopramide
Amitriptyline	Estrogens (in males)	Metoprolol
Carbamazepine	Finasteride	Nelfinavir
Chlorpromazine	Fluoxetine	Paroxetine
Chlorthalidone	Fluvoxamine	Phenytoin
Cimetidine (high dose)	Fosamprenavir	Progesterone
Cisplatin	Haloperidol	Propranolol
Citalopram	Hydrochlorothiazide	Ritonavir
Clofibrate	Imipramine	Saquinavir
Clomipramine	Indinavir	Sertraline
Clonidine	Ketoconazole	Spironolactone
Desipramine	Lithium	(larger doses)
Diazepam	Methadone	Tamoxifen
Digoxin	Methyldopa	Timolol

D | Medications That Can Cause Erectile Problems

Acetazolamide	Desipramine	Methyldopa
Amitriptyline	Digoxin	Metoprolol
Atenolol	Haloperidol	Nadolol
Baclofen	Hydralazine	Naproxen
Carbamazepine	Hydrochlorothiazide	Phenytoin
Carvedilol	Imipramine	Prazosin
Chlorpromazine	Finasteride	Progesterone
Chlorthalidone	Fluoxetine	Propranolol
Cimetidine	Fluphenazine	Sertraline
Citalopram	Fluvoxamine	Sotalol
Clofibrate	Labetalol	Spironolactone
Clomipramine	Lithium	Timolol
Clonidine	Methadone	Venlafaxine

E | Medications That Can Lead to Male Breast Enlargement

Amitriptyline	Etomidate	Penicillamine
Anabolic steroids	Finasteride	Phenytoin
Androgens	Flutamide	Pravastatin
Captopril	Haloperidol	Prochloperazine
Cimetidine	Isoniazid	Ranitidine
Cisplatin	Ketoconazole	Spironolactone
Diazepam	Methyldopa	Thioridazine
Digoxin	Metoclopramide	Verapamil
Enalapril	Metronidazole	
Estrogens	Omeprazole	

F | Some Medications That Interact with Birth Control Pills/Patch/Ring

Many antibiotics interfere with hormonal birth control. Use an additional method of birth control during and for the rest of the cycle following antibiotic use.

DRUG	EFFECT
Acetaminophen	may need higher dose for pain relief
Alcohol	possible increased alcohol effect
Amitriptyline	increased effects and side effects
Ampicillin	possible decreased contraceptive effect
ASA	may need higher dose for pain relief and anti-inflammatory effect
Atenolol	possible increased drug effect
Caffeine	increased caffeine effect
Carbamazepine	increased risk of pregnancy, increased breakthrough bleeding
Clofibrate	weakened lipid-lowering effect
Corticosteroids	increased steroid effect and side effects
Cyclosporine	possible increased cyclosporine side effects due to higher cyclosporine levels
Diazepam	increased sedative effect
Fosamprenavir	increased risk of pregnancy
Indinavir	increased risk of pregnancy
Insulin	may require more insulin
Laxatives	increased breakthrough bleeding, increased risk of pregnancy
Levothyroxine	may need higher dose of thyroid medicine
Lorazepam	both increased and decreased drowsiness reported
Metoprolol	possible increased effects
Morphine	decreased morphine levels (possible decreased painkilling)
Nadolol	possible increased effects
Nelfinavir	increased risk of pregnancy
Nevirapine	increased risk of pregnancy
Oxazepam	both increased and decreased drowsiness reported
Phenobarbital	increased risk of pregnancy
Phenytoin	increased breakthrough bleeding, increased risk of pregnancy, increased side effects of phenytoin
Prednisone	increased prednisone effects
Propranolol	possible increased effects
Rifampin	increased risk of pregnancy
Ritonavir	increased risk of pregnancy
Sirolimus	possible increased side effects of sirolimus due to higher sirolimus levels
Tacrolimus	possible increased side effects of tacrolimus due to higher tacrolimus levels
Tetracycline	possible decreased contraceptive effect
Theophylline	increased theophylline side effects
Thyroxine	see Levothyroxine
Tolbutamide	hypoglycemia
Trimethoprim-sulfamethoxazole	increased estrogen levels (may experience some nausea or other side effects)
Valproate	no effect
Vitamin C (1 gr or more per day)	increased estrogen blood levels, therefore increased birth control pill side effects
Warfarin	decreased anticoagulant effect

G Some Over-the-Counter (OTC)/Prescription Drug Interactions		
OTC	**PRESCRIPTION**	**EFFECT**
Acetaminophen (Tylenol®, Tempra®)	Carbamazepine Phenobarbital Phenytoin Rifampin Valproic Acid Zidovudine (AZT)	Risk of liver damage with repeated use

Bone marrow toxicity—rare |
Antacids (Maalox®, Mylanta®, Tums®)	Ciprofloxacin Tetracyclines Digoxin Phenytoin Ranitidine/cimetidine Corticosteroids	Antacids can cause decreased absorption and therefore less drug activity
Antihistamines: Diphenhydramine (Benadryl®) or Nytol®	Sedatives: Liazepam (Valium®) or Lorazepam Narcotic painkillers (e.g., Codeine, Hydromorphone, Morphine)	Sedation, confusion, falls
Antinauseants: Meclizine/ Dimenhydrynate	Phenytoin Sedatives Narcotic painkillers	Increased levels and side effects
ASA (Aspirin®)	Warfarin (any ASA) Valproic Acid (regular use of ASA) Prednisone (regular use of ASA)	Bleeding Risk of liver damage Increased chance of ulcers
Cold remedies containing Pseudoephedrine (e.g., Benylin®, Sudafed®)	Atenolol Carvedilol Metoprolol Nadolol Labetolol Salbutamol	Increased side effects

Tremor, palpitations |
| Cough syrups with Dextromethorphan | Amiodarone Fluoxetine Quinidine | Increased side effects of cough remedy |
| NSAIDS: Ibuprofen (Advil®, Motrin®) or Naproxen (Aleve®) | Warfarin ASA Lithium | Risk of bleeding Stomach ulcers, pain, kidney damage Increased side effects |

H Street Drugs and Their Possible Effect on Sexual Function				
Drug	Decreases Sexual Interest	Erectile Difficulties	Inhibits Orgasm	Delays or Prevents Ejaculation
Alcohol	Yes	Yes		
Amphetamines	Yes	Yes	Yes	Yes
Cocaine	Yes		Yes	Yes
Diazepam	Yes			Yes
Heroin	Yes	Yes	Yes	Yes
Marijuana	Yes	Yes		
Nitrous Oxide		Yes		
PCP (chronic use)	Yes	Yes		Yes

I Possible Effects of Drinking Alcohol When Taking Medication	
DRUG	**EFFECT**
Acetaminophen	liver damage with large amounts or frequent drinking and routine use of acetaminophen
Amitriptyline	reduced alertness and attention
Antihistamines	drowsiness, difficulty concentrating, slow reflexes
ASA (Aspirin®)	stomach bleeding
Bethanechol	increased alcohol absorption, feels as though you've had more to drink
Buproprion	increased risk of seizures
Captopril	dizziness, sleepiness, low blood pressure
Carbamazepine	increased sleepiness, dizziness, confusion
Celecoxib	nausea, stomach pain, stomach bleeding
Cephalosporin	decreased blood pressure, antibiotics, nausea and vomiting flushing, headache, fast heart rate, cramps
Chlorpromazine	makes uncontrollable movements (EPS) worse
Cimetidine	no effect, but if you have an ulcer, can make it worse
Cisapride	increased alcohol absorption, feels as though you've had more to drink
Clobazam	slowed breathing, sleepiness, confusion **death**
Clonazepam	slowed breathing, sleepiness, confusion **death**
Clonidine	sleepiness, dizziness, confusion
Codeine	slowed breathing, sleepiness, confusion **death**

I Possible Effects of Drinking Alcohol When Taking Medication	
DRUG	**EFFECT**
Cyclosporine	heavy drinking can raise cyclosporine levels
Benzodiazepines	slowed breathing, sleepiness, confusion, slow reflexes **death**
Didanosine	increased amount of alcohol in the blood pancreatitis (very painful)
Domperidone	increased alcohol absorption
Enalapril	low blood pressure, dizziness, sleepiness
Fluconazole	may be the same as ketoconazole (see below)
Fluvoxamine	increased blood levels of fluvoxamine, decreased alertness and attention
Glyburide	increased risk of hypoglycemia
Haloperidol	makes uncontrollable movements (EPS) worse
Indomethacin	damage to lining of stomach
Insulin	low blood sugar (especially if you don't eat) long-term signs of high blood sugar drinking in moderation may have little effect
Ketoconazole	sweating, redness, nausea
Lithium	increased lithium levels reduced alertness and attention
Lorazepam	slowed breathing, sleepiness, confusion **death**
Metformin	lactic acidosis (not a good thing) hypoglycemia
Methotrexate	liver damage
Metronidazole	decreased blood pressure, nausea and vomiting, flushing headache, fast heart rate, cramps
Nifedipine	increased nifedipine levels, low blood pressure, dizziness
Olanzapine	increased uncontrollable movements (EPS), confusion, dizziness
Phenytoin	lowers blood levels if drinking a lot or often, sleepiness, dizziness, confusion
Propranolol	may lower amount in bloodstream

I	Possible Effects of Drinking Alcohol When Taking Medication
DRUG	**EFFECT**
Risperidone	increased uncontrollable movements (EPS), confusion, dizziness
Sirolimus	heavy drinking may increase sirolimus levels
Sotalol	decreased blood pressure
Tacrolimus	heavy drinking may increase tacrolimus levels
Topiramate	dizziness, confusion
Valproic acid	sleepiness, dizziness, confusion

J	Possible Effects of Tobacco Use with Medication
DRUG	**EFFECT**
Amiodarone	decreased effect
Amitriptyline	decreased effect
Amlodipine	raised blood pressure and heart rate
Chlorpromazine	decreased effect
Cimetidine	increased nicotine effects, decreased cimetidine effect
Clozapine	decreased effect
Diazepam	decreased effect
Haloperidol	decreased effect
Insulin	need more insulin takes longer for it to work
Fluphenazine	decreased effect
Fluvoxamine	may need more medication
Olanzapine	decreased levels
Propranolol	decreased effect
Ranitidine	increased nicotine levels
Theophylline	decreased effect
Vitamins C and B12	decreased levels
Warfarin	may change warfarin levels and INR (up or down)

K	Possible Effects of Marijuana Use with Medication
DRUG	**EFFECT**
Amiodarone	with frequent use, may make the drug leave your body more quickly, decreasing its effect
Amitriptyline	very fast heart beat, mood swings, hallucinations, confusion
Amlodipine	dizziness, fast heart rate
Amphetamines	increased heart rate, increased shakiness
Antihistamines	increased drowsiness
Benzodiazepines	increased drowsiness
Carbamazepine	frequent marijuana use can change carbamazepine levels; sleepiness, dizziness, confusion
Chlorpromazine	severe dizziness, confusion, difficulty thinking; decreased amount of chlorpromazine in your body
Clomipramine	very fast heart rate, dizziness, mood swings, hallucinations, confusion
Cyclosporine	raised cyclosporine levels, possible cyclosporine toxicity
Fosamprenavir	stronger marijuana effects
Indinavir	lower levels of indinavir
Insulin	small to moderate use will probably have no effect; frequent use may increase need for insulin
Lithium	increased lithium levels
Nelfinavir	lower levels of nelfinavir, stronger marijuana effect
Phenytoin	decreased effect of phenytoin
Propranolol	probably not affected by marijuana use although little data available
Ritonavir	stronger marijuana effect
Saquinavir	stronger marijuana effect
Sirolimus	raised sirolimus levels, possibly sirolimus toxicity
Tacrolimus	raised tacrolimus levels, possibly tacrolimus toxicity
Theophylline	decreased levels in bloodstream
Topiramate	can worsen sleepiness, dizziness and confusion that is a side effect of topiramate
Valproic acid	increased sleepiness, dizziness, confusion, decreased alertness
Warfarin	may change warfarin levels, and INR may go up or down; if smoking more than once a week, get INR checked more often

L Possible Effects of Cocaine Use with Medication	
DRUG	**EFFECT**
Amitriptyline	makes cocaine levels higher
Amlodipine	high blood pressure and rapid heart beat from cocaine can counteract medication effect
Chlorpromazine	may increase risk of EPS (uncontrollable movements)
Haloperidol	may increase risk of EPS
Loxapine	may increase risk of EPS
Olanzapine	may increase risk of EPS
Pimozide	may increase risk of EPS
Propranolol	covers up some of the effects of cocaine, so dangerously high levels of cocaine can be reached; stroke or heart attack, death can result
Quetiapine	increased risk of EPS
Risperidone	increased risk of EPS, high temperature
Sotalol	very high blood pressure, rapid heart beat, heart attack, stroke, death
Trazodone	painful erection that won't go away

M Possible Effects of Amphetamine (Including Ecstasy) Use with Medication	
DRUG	**EFFECT**
Amitriptyline	makes amphetamine levels higher
Amlodipine	fast heart beat, high blood pressure
Chlorpromazine	increased levels of amphetamines
Citalopram	high fever, nausea, very high blood pressure, **death**
Clomipramine	amphetamines stay in body for longer, increased effects
Clonidine	**death**
Delavirdine	very high levels of speed or ecstasy in your blood can lead to overdose or death
Fluvoxamine	high fever, high blood pressure, heart problems, **death**
Fosamprenavir	very high levels of speed or ecstasy in your blood can lead to overdose or **death**
Indinavir	very high levels of speed or ecstasy in your blood can lead to overdose or **death**
Nelfinavir	very high levels of speed or ecstasy in your blood can lead to overdose or **death**
Paroxetine	high fever, high blood pressure, heart problems, **death**
Propranolol	high blood pressure, fast heart beat, heart attack, stroke, **death**
Ritonavir	very high levels of speed or ecstasy in your blood, can lead to overdose or **death**
Saquinavir	very high levels of speed or ecstasy in your blood, can lead to overdose or **death**
Sertraline	high fever, high blood pressure, heart problems, **death**
Sotalol	high blood pressure, fast heart beat, heart attack, stroke, **death**

N	Drugs Which, If Combined with PCP, Can Lead to Seizures, High Blood Pressure, High Temperature or Muscle Destruction		
Delavirdine	Indinavir	Stavudine
Didanosine	Lamivudine	Zidovudine
Efavirenz	Ritonavir	
Fosamprenavir	Saquinavir	

O	Possible Effects of LSD Use with Medication
Abacavir	extreme fear, anxiety, flashbacks
Amitriptyline	feelings of terror, bad trip, prolonged trip
Citalopram	bad trip or decreased LSD effect
Clomipramine	extreme fear, bad trip, prolonged trip
Fluoxetine	bad trip, extreme fear, prolonged trip
Fosamprenavir	extreme fear, anxiety, flashbacks
Paroxetine	bad trip, extreme fear, prolonged trip
Sertraline	bad trip, extreme fear, prolonged trip, flashbacks
Trazodone	bad trip, extreme fear, prolonged trip

P	Other Combinations to Avoid		

Any heart or blood pressure medication and mushrooms or cocaine

Any seizure medication and cocaine or amphetamines

Antidepressants and caffeine

Amitriptyline and heroin, codeine or morphine

Amlodipine and heroin, codeine or morphine

Chlorpromazine and heroin, codeine or morphine

Cimetidine and benzodiazepines

Clobazam and heroin, codeine or morphine; ketamine

Clomipramine and heroin, codeine or morphine;

benzodiazepines

Clonazepam and heroin, codeine or morphine; ketamine; benzodiazepines

Codeine and ketamine; heroin, codeine or morphine; benzodiazepines

Cyclosporine and heroin

Delavirdine and valium; heroin, codeine or morphine; ketamine

Diazepam and ketamine

Digoxin and benzodiazepines

Efavirenz and ketamine or benzodiazepines

Fluoxetine and codeine

Fosmprenavir and ketamine

Indinavir and ketamine

or benzodiazepines

Itraconazole and benzodiazepines

Lamivudine and ketamine

Lithium and caffeine (four or more colas or coffees per day) or ketamine

Nelfinavir and ketamine or benzodiazepines

Nevirapine and ketamine or benzodiazepines

Ritonavir and ketamine

Saquinavir and ketamine

Stavudine and ketamine

Tacrolimus and heroin

Zidovudine and ketamine

Q Medications That Can Cause Skin Sensitivity to the Sun		
Acetazolamide	Ciprofloxacin	Ketoconazole
Alprazolam	Clozapine	Lamotrigine
Amantadine	Coal tar	Lisinopril
Amiodarone	Diclofenac	Methotrexate
Amitriptyline	Diltiazem	Minocycline
Amlodipine	Enalapril	Naproxen
Azathioprine	Fosinopril	Trimethoprim-
Captopril	Furosemide	sulfamethoxazole
Carbamazepine	Ganciclovir	Valacyclovir
Carvedilol	Hydrochlorothiazide	Valproic acid
Cetirizine	Ibuprofen	Voriconazole
Chlorothiazide	Isotretinoin	
Chlorpromazine	Itraconazole	

GENERAL INFORMATION

www.aboutkidshealth.ca A comprehensive site with an A-to-Z listing of conditions, an interactive animated anatomy atlas and much more. Although quite a bit of it is aimed at parents and smaller kids, it is worth a look.

IBD Academy is a free app (Apple and Android) that lets you monitor your symptoms and keep track of your medical information. It will graph your mood and do lots of other helpful stuff. If you have inflammatory bowel disease, you should check it out.

www.kidshealth.org/teen TeensHealth lists a whole bunch of diseases and gives details about them.

www.lehman.cuny.edu/faculty/jfleitas/bandaides/contteen.html This really long URL takes you to the Band-Aides and Blackboard site, which uses personal storytelling and art to communicate the experience of having a chronic health condition.

http://mssociety.ca/en/help/booklets.htm On this page you will find several free downloadable booklets for youth, as well as (in the Managing Symptoms section) an excellent booklet about multiple sclerosis and sex, mainly written for adults.

www.mymedschedule.com Both a website and free app (Apple and Android) that helps you plot and track your meds. You can print off a schedule (and even choose to include pics of the different meds) and have it remind you to take your meds.

www.nhtsa.dot.gov An American site for the National Highway Traffic Safety Administration. There is a lot of very technical information here, but there is also quite a bit on adapting vehicles.

www.osteoporosis.ca This easy-to-use site has a calcium calculator: you select the amount of foods you eat from the list and it tells you how much calcium you are getting.

www.sickkids.ca/good2go   This site has several tools to help teens with their transition from pediatric to adult care, including a readiness checklist and a parent tip sheet that you can print off for your parents.

www.sickkids.ca/myhealthpassport   This free program lets you print a wallet-sized card with all your important health information. Choose from one (or more) of 50 templates, fill in your info and print. You can also e-mail a copy to yourself or someone else. Great in a medical emergency or when you are seeing a new health care practitioner. You can laminate it (laminators are often found at bus stations and drug stores), or just use clear packing tape.

SPORTS

www.ncpad.org   The National Center on Physical Activity and Disability has lots of information, both general and specific, for a number of disabilities.

Paralympic Committees

www.napcosa.co.za   South Africa

www.paralympic.ca   Canada

www.paralympic.org   The International Paralympic Committee has affiliated paralympic committees in many countries. Each of their sites will have a listing of sports organizations in their country and often other information.

www.europaralympic.org   Europe

www.paralympic.org.au   Australia

www.paralympics.org.nz   New Zealand

www.paralympics.org.uk   United Kingdom

www2.teamusa.org/US-Paralympics.aspx   United States

TRAVEL

www.gimponthego.com   Gimp on the Go has travel tips and reviews, particularly helpful for people with mobility issues.

www.independentliving.org   The Independent Living Institute has a good website in general. The Vacation Home part of the site lists accessible homes available to be traded for a home in another country for a vacation.

www.sath.org   The Society for Accessible Travel & Hospitality has a Travel Tips section for people who are deaf, autistic, arthritic, diabetic, blind or have mobility issues. It also provides information on accessibility and several airlines and hotels. The Resources section lists tour operators that specialize in different types of disabilities. The Need to Know section has information on going through airport security.

SEX AND GENDER
Where to Buy Sex Toys Online
Canada: **www.comeasyouare.com**   The store in Toronto is wheelchair accessible and has helpful staff. Sales are available online and the site has lots of good info.

U.S.: **www.goodvibes.com**   Good Vibrations is the grandmother of cool, aware sex-toy stores. Physically located in San Francisco, it is home to the Antique Vibrator Museum.

Europe: **www.lovehoney.co.uk**   Lovehoney doesn't have the same activist cred as Good Vibrations and Come as You Are, but it is known for its excellent customer service.

Publications
Sexuality and Cerebral Palsy is available online at **www.ofcp. ca/pdf/book/sexuality_book.pdf** or can be ordered for $5 as a print edition from the Ontario Federation for Cerebral Palsy (416) 244-9686

The Ultimate Guide to Sex and Disability by Miriam Kaufman, Cory Silverberg and Fran Odette. Cleis Press, 2007.

Websites
www.comeasyouare.com/default/index.cfm/sex-tips/sex-and-disability   Come as You Are is a Canadian sex-toy store that has information about making sex toys accessible and links to other sex and disability-related sites.

www.goaskalice.columbia.edu   Go Ask Alice! is a terrific site with questions and answers about sex (almost anything you can think of), emotional issues and health. You can post questions.

www.isna.org   The Intersex Society of North America site offers information about and support for people with a variety of intersex conditions (such as androgen insensitivity and CAH).

www.scarleteen.com   Scarleteen has information and discussions about many aspects of sex, contraception and relationships.

www.sexuality.about.com   Everything you might want to know about sex, including a great page on adapting sex toys, plus other sex and disability information.

www.lehman.cuny.edu/faculty/jfleitas/bandaides/contteen. html   The Band-Aides and Blackboards website offers personal stories, links to info, poems and art.

www.sexuality.org   This site is filled with excellent information about sex resources in print and online.

www.sexetc.org   Sex, Etc. is a site run by teens with information about sex, abortion and health.

Index